A FORK IN THE ROAD...

An inspiring journey of how ancient
Solfeggio frequencies are empowering
personal and planetary transformation!

David Hulse, D.D

AuthorHouse™
1663 Liberty Drive
Bloomington, IN 47403
www.authorhouse.com
Phone: 1-800-839-8640

© 2009 David Hulse, D.D. All rights reserved.

No part of this book may be reproduced, stored in a retrieval system, or transmitted by any means without the written permission of the author.

First published by AuthorHouse 8/27/2009

ISBN: 978-1-4389-5791-3 (sc)

Printed in the United States of America
Bloomington, Indiana

This book is printed on acid-free paper.

TABLE OF CONTENTS

Dedication iv
Acknowledgements vii
Introduction viii
From Fundamentalist Preacher to Tuning Forks viii

PART ONE – MY JOURNEY 1

CHAPTER ONE - MY FIRST SPIRITUAL EXPERIENCE 1

Light Experience Changes My Life Forever 3
Harmonic Convergence 3
Misery In Memphis 4
The Dark Abyss 6
The Illusion 7
Principle of Synchronicity 8
Hit By Lightning! 9
A Sacred Sound Within Me 11
I Had To Get Real 12
Angry at God 13
A Course In Miracles 16

CHAPTER TWO - THE DARKNESS 18

Take Another Look 19
Good and Very Good 20
A Course in Miracles and the Unified Field 21
Everything is Relationship! 22
Second Great Spiritual Experience – The Life Review Vision 23
A New Energy is Coming 24
A Free Will Planet 26
The 144,000 28
The Frequency to Repair DNA 29

CHAPTER THREE – JUST INTONATION & 12-TONE EQUAL TEMPERAMENT 32

CHAPTER FOUR - HOW I FOUND OUT ABOUT THE ANCIENT SOLFEGGIO SCALE 36

    How Dr. Puleo Deciphered the Six Frequencies.......... 36
    Professor Willi Apel.. 38
    What was I to Do with These Forks? 39
    Playing with the Tuning Forks....................................... 40
    Development of SomaEnergetics Techniques.............. 43
    Third Vision: The Missing Stones 44
    Vibrational Fields 47
    A Recipe for the Universe... 48
    Realizing Our Ultimate Potential as Human Beings..... 48
    Where Are the Lightworkers? 50

CHAPTER FIVE— ENERGY WORK AND SOMAENERGETICS... 51

    Fifth Dimensional Energy.. 51
    The Solfeggio and Six Precious Metals 54
    Energy Dynamics of the Vesica Piscis......................... 54
    The Causes of Aches & Pains 56
    The Secret within the Solfeggio Syllables.................... 59
    Hidden Meanings in the Frequencies 60
    The Frequencies and the Chakras................................ 61
    SomaEnergetics Frequencies.. 63
    Level II Workshops 65
    Level III Workshops – Teacher Certification 66
    Purchasing Tuning Forks.. 67

CHAPTER SIX - INTENTION, IMAGINATION & INTUITION... 68

    Imagination 68
    Intention 69
    Intuition 70

PART TWO – THE SCIENCE OF SOUND........................74

CHAPTER SEVEN - MUSICAL SYSTEMS 74

    Consonance 75
    The Hand of God Tunes the World............................... 76

The Ut Note? 77
A Hertz Makes A Difference 79
Your Secret Ear 80
Finding the Key to the Universe 81

CHAPTER EIGHT - THE SCIENCE OF SOUND & VIBRATIONAL HEALING 83

Alice Bailey 85
Cathie Guzette 86
Guiliana Conforto 86
Dale Pond 87
The "C" Family Gene 87
Geopathic Stress 88
Royal Raymond Rife 89
Chladni Sand Figures 90
Hans Jenny 90
Dr. John Beaulieu 91
Dr. Andrew Weil 92
Entrainment 93
Process 94

CHAPTER 9: DNA RESEARCH 96

Deoxyribonucleic Acid – DNA 96
The Dance of Shiva 98
Living In The Field 99
Turning the Switch On 100
Misspelled DNA 102
Let Us Move On 104

APPENDIX A 107

WORKS CITED 108

WEBSITES CITED 112

Dedication

This book is for Bea Hulse, who was not only a great mother, but also my best friend.

We will not suffer the negative radiation, or excessive ultra-violet radiations that will bombard places of the earth for we will inhabit the safe zones at the time of the great geo-physical upheavals. Those who are not protected against the radiation will fulfill once again the ancient pre-Aztec saying which speaks of 'Those who were carried away by the Sun's rays into destruction.' […]The thought adjusters are now correcting and repairing our blood crystallization levels of ionized consciousness through FREQUENCY ATTUNEMENT.

Key 213:31-33
From *The Keys of Enoch* by J.J. Hurtak *(1977)*

Acknowledgements

Several editors and friends have assisted in shaping this book including but not limited to Linda Bloomfield, Marcy Cheek, Betty Onyett, Phadia Adams, Tobie Saad, Sarla Matsumura, Sue McSherry, Randall Loop and Tim Leach. My thanks to these individuals for sharing their talents and energy to make this book what it has become.

I would like to also offer thanks to all of my teachers who are too numerous to mention. This is a book of speculative thought. What is written here is simply my personal version of truth. I have borrowed freely from the great ideas of others and I do not claim special or unusual insight.

I will share information from other authors that was helpful in this journey of discovery. I have given my best effort to properly crediting these individuals. In the event I have left anyone out, please contact me so that proper credit may be given where it is due.

This is a summary of my six decades on the planet. My purpose is to share the realizations I have had on my personal path of growth and to present concepts that might stimulate new ideas. Scientific inaccuracies in this book are unintentional.

I also would like to clarify that the word *man* comes from the most ancient language on the planet, Sanskrit, from the word *manus*, which means to think. The term is sometimes used in this book when it appears in others' direct quotes that were written before the words man or mankind became associated with gender awareness and inclusiveness. However, the over-all understanding of the word *man* is to include all of humankind, male and female.

David Hulse
September 2009

Introduction

> "When you come to a fork in the road, take it."
> Yogi Berra

From Fundamentalist Preacher to Tuning Forks

I stand here listening to the sounds of meditative music floating from the speakers of the CD player while the aroma of essential oils and incense permeate my senses. I am aware that I am standing over someone on a massage table in need of healing. I cannot help but reflect on my journey – from the southern gospel piano player, singer, and fundamentalist preacher of my youth who held a bible and prayed to Jesus, to the energy worker who holds a tuning fork for the same purpose of healing through aligning energies and balancing chakras.

In my travels across the country, the question asked most frequently is how I went from being a fundamentalist preacher to being a developer of healing techniques using tuning forks. This book is the story of that journey. I feel honored yet humbled to be among those rising to the call to facilitate the new 5th Dimensional energy coming into our third dimensional time/space continuum.

Come with me as we journey step by step through my search for answers. After looking at what I refer to in this book as my Fork in the Road, a new truth was born – a truth that provides answers for the Spirit, Mind, and Body. I will share information concerning self-healing using sound, vibration, and frequencies that can clear, cleanse, balance, and focus our lives in all its forms. The ancient Solfeggio frequencies are part of a process that can assist us in creating the possibility of lives without stress, illness, and sickness. Together we will go to the cutting edge of scientific discoveries regarding sound and healing.

David Hulse, D.D.

This book is also a call for Lightworkers to gather in this crucial time of change and transformation on the planet. Join me and others who do not live in fear of the future. Just tune your inner ear and listen to these wonderful new ideas as I share the techniques of working with sound and, more specifically, the Solfeggio tuning forks.

My hope is that we can all find the harmonics of our own individual music, and that through this process we will be enabled to live balanced lives.

PART ONE – MY JOURNEY

CHAPTER ONE - MY FIRST SPIRITUAL EXPERIENCE

At age 16 I had the first of three major spiritual experiences – a profound mystical experience that changed my life forever. I lived in Tulsa Oklahoma and played the piano for the church I attended. One day it came to my attention that the church down the street from ours was having an old-fashioned revival meeting. As the meeting grew, they had erected a big tent to accommodate the large crowd.

I became very curious about what they were doing and what was causing all the excitement. The people who went to my church told me not to go. I entertained the idea of not going, but I felt this *pull* I could not deny. Being a Sagittarian, I could not help but venture out of my religious box into uncharted territory, as Sagittarians are known for their insatiable curiosity.

One night, very deliberately and quietly, I snuck in through the back of the tent. So much for my efforts; the man who was preaching saw me and kept looking in my direction. He was starting an altar call – a time during the revival when people are invited to come forward and make a decision to serve God with their lives. This preacher saw me and asked me to come forward. I felt drawn to get out of my seat and walk towards him. I made my way through the crowd, not really understanding why I was going as I felt I had already given my life to God. I continued to make my way up to the front when the minister holding the revival spoke to me and said, "Receive God's Spirit." As soon as he said that, I was so consumed with such a massive amount of energy that I fell to the floor – literally "slain in the spirit," as we called it in those days. *Immediately* within my mind's eye, I saw a great Light. The Light was alive, living, pulsing with life and color and I felt feelings beyond my normal perception. While it is hard to find the words to describe the experience, I do remember feeling very secure, very safe. I did not see a form, but at that time, I perceived the Light to be Jesus. I thought I heard "the Lord" speaking directly to me at the time. Upon reflection, I feel it was more of "a knowing." The voice seemed to say, "My son, go and gather twelve yellow roses, bring them back and present them to me."

Up to this point in my spiritual path and career, I had never had any kind of experience like this; this was incredible. I remember feeling so honored to be able to gather the roses. As the inner vision continued, I felt a huge impetus to fulfill this request of Jesus. I began to walk through the streets searching for a florist shop. I found a shop, but when I went inside my heart sank, as all of the yellow roses in the shop were wilting and dying. I thought to myself, I could not give these sadly wilted roses to the Lord. In the vision, I remember feeling despair in my search and I was about to give up when my eye caught the most perfect yellow rosebud in the midst of all of the other flowers in the shop, and I purchased it. I went down the street and found another florist shop. There I found another perfect yellow rosebud, and I purchased it. I continued walking through the streets, finding more and more florist shops and purchasing each perfect yellow rose until I had a total of twelve.

I took the roses back and presented them to the Light. Internally, I heard the Light say to me:

As you have gone and gathered these roses for me, so shall you go and gather the fragments of Truth contained in all of the major centers of information in the world today. From various religions, philosophies, and even science, all contain a certain part of the Truth. No one has all of the answers or some type of exclusivity on Truth. The Truth will never be in only one place and under the control of any one group of people. The Truth is free and expanding and forever being revealed. As you gathered the yellow roses, you have gathered parts of The Eternal Wisdom. Now take these to my people, for as you have done this unto me, so have you done this unto them.

Again, this was truly a profound experience unlike anything I had ever experienced. I later learned that yellow is the color of Wisdom. The Greek word *Sofia* means Wisdom, represented as the color yellow, or the *golden* light. This golden light of wisdom will reappear in the third major vision of my life, which we will explore later in this book.

Light Experience Changes My Life Forever

It was not too long after this first spiritual experience that I began my ministry at seventeen years old. At that time, which was the early1960's, most preachers in the North American south and southwest were preaching that Jesus was coming soon. As an impressionable teenager whose innocent heart was deeply touched by the good news about how to end the misery and suffering in the world, I wanted to tell the world that Jesus could take away all of their problems. Nonetheless, I did not see where preaching that Jesus was coming soon would encourage people to be responsible for their lives. They would just sit on the pew and wait for Jesus to come. This perception caused me to create a message that diverged from the mainstream at that time. My new thoughts and inspirations were not widely accepted. I preached the good news that Christ in us was the hope of Glory. That glory was the total salvation – spirit, soul and body - NOW. This message later became that Christ in us IS the Glory and that we are the Glory of God on earth.

Harmonic Convergence

By the mid to late 80's, I felt a part of something larger than myself. When I heard about the Harmonic Convergence in 1987, I asked all the staff and local friends of my ministry to join me at 5 AM to hold hands in a park and express gratitude and availability for the new energy coming into the earth. They thought it was a strange request, but they did it anyway. During the expression of gratitude, I felt a shift.

I knew beyond understanding that I was about to enter a new adventure – another fork in the road of life.

The Harmonic Convergence was a loosely organized spiritual event, which occurred on August 16 and 17, 1987. Groups of people gathered in various sacred sites and mystical places all over the world with the intention to usher in a new era. The date was based primarily on the Mayan calendar, but also on interpretations of European and Asian astrology.

An interesting explanation of the Harmonic Convergence is offered by Barbara Marciniak, in *Earth: Pleiadian Keys to the Living Library*. She writes that the Harmonic Convergence was a primary event, "an occurrence that is registered within the prime webwork in the corridors of time as a pivotal juncture around which all of reality transits. It can be considered an event that is a turning point for the domain in which it transpires." (1994, 191)

I continued on a ministerial path until November 1988 when I found myself in Memphis, Tennessee and I thought my ministry was at an end. Little did I understand at that time that the ending in Memphis was just a new beginning. Like the phoenix rising from its ashes, the beginning of my journey using tuning forks to bring health and healing to our planet came at what seemed to be the end of everything in my life.

Misery In Memphis

In November of 1988 I was in Memphis, Tennessee ministering to a group who had heard that I preached up a storm and could sing and play a mean ragtime piano in black gospel style. In some religious circles – more particularly, the Christian Pentecostals – it is believed that a good preacher was one who could get everyone awake and excited, clapping their hands and shouting "Amen." A good preacher could whip the crowd into a frenzy of emotionalism and make them feel happy. A good preacher could help a person forget all his or her troubles, at least while at church.

Today, it is common knowledge that the physical body can be stimulated in various ways to produce serotonin; thus elevating our moods and helping us to feel happy. Back then, we did not attribute this to serotonin, though we did know we could get the physical body to wake up, get involved, just by singing a song over and over and by clapping our hands. The same result happened when the preachers would preach at the top of their lungs with lots of gestures and dramatic emphasis, and the congregation took part with loud "Amens" and "Praise the Lords."

The basic message that I preached in those days was called the *Manifested Sons of God* message. I accepted the invitation to speak in Memphis because I had spoken to other groups around the country who shared that same idea that centered on how to become a fully matured son or daughter of God. I emphasized that we were not to continue to be little children, sitting in the high chair, needing Mom or Dad to feed us. That high chair was the pew in which we sat every Sunday, being spoon-fed by the preacher, being told what to think and what to believe. I explained to them that we should begin to take responsibility for making our own decisions about what to do, where to go, and what to believe, as well as how to embrace maturity and become an adult son or daughter of God. We were to become independent, self-sufficient, and ready to both lead and teach others – by giving them a word of encouragement or revelation to help them along their path to do the same. Looking back at my experiences, I now realize that salvation is not a one-time event. It is a process of discovering our innate wisdom and learning to rely on that guidance within.

I usually did not go to traditional, structured, denominational churches because I did not have the right credentials. An elderly woman had originally ordained me up in the hills of

Oklahoma. She "felt" that I had been "called of God," and she sent me forth with Ordination Papers issued by the congregation of her church. There was not a category for the type of preacher I was, one independent of organized religion. I traveled around the country, preaching mostly in people's homes, or sometimes, if enough people showed up, someone would rent a room in a hotel or lodge. We also had revivals in those days, sometimes lasting weeks.

I knew I could go and speak in Memphis, probably saying things I had spoken dozens of times, many of those times without really being present in the moment. Most non-denominational fundamentalist preachers, like me, preached with an "Anointing of the Holy Spirit," which meant we were channeling from our higher selves. I would prepare material and be knowledgeable about the scriptures, but when it came time to give the message, I would give myself over to the Holy Spirit and be available to share a fresh word of revelation and minister directly to the needs of the people through words of wisdom and words of knowledge.

After so many years of being in the ministry, I had learned how to preach a good message from a vast storehouse of information and knowledge I had gathered, gleaned, and stored away in my brain. I could reference just about anything I needed to make a point. Words, like fireworks shot into the sky to dazzle and daze the congregation. I would take them from the mundane and misery of their lives and give them a moment of excitement and even personal revelation. I knew I could go to Memphis that day and not disappoint them. At the very least, I knew I could get them going in their physical bodies to release a lot of energy and make them *feel* happy. They would think I was great.

The Dark Abyss

Yet, tragically, I did not think I was great. Inside, I was destitute. I felt bare, empty, and lacking. In the many months before this engagement, whenever I got up to minister, I would look out, and it seemed that I was looking into a dark abyss, emptiness, a vast nothingness – a void. I kept thinking, "This is the end of my ministry." I seemed to be preaching the same concepts and saying the same words I had learned from external sources that no longer resonated at each service. I believed in my heart that I was speaking the truth, but I didn't see any evidence of it in the lives of the people who listened to me and, most of all, I didn't see it in my own life. I really did not know what I was going to do. I was literally dying inside and I was miserable in Memphis.

Adding to my immediate distress, during my stay I was in a motel in one of the worst parts of Memphis. It was so bad that a sign had been posted in the room cautioning guests to keep the door locked. I did not have a car, so I could not drive to a movie. I could not even go out for a walk. I was stuck in that awful room by myself. There was nowhere to go, nothing to do, nothing to believe in, no one to comfort me, and no answers to anything.

The Illusion

Before I go further, let me tell you I have since learned that we are never really in that state. It is an illusion, outward circumstances created by certain types of vibrational thoughts that appear to be miserable, but are just vibrations and are subject to being changed in an instant – in the twinkling of an eye – by any new and immediate intention, thought, or desire. I have also learned that the benevolent Universe has all things already prepared for us for any eventuality beyond what we can possibly conceive or think. The Universe is prepared to manifest any intention, is prepared for any thought, prepared to bring to pass any desire of our hearts in any moment of our lives. It does not matter how desolate, delirious, destitute, or totally hopeless we feel. It only appears that way. Our situation really is NEVER desolate, destitute, or hopeless. That is the illusion. If you remember anything from this reading, remember this – it might change your life.

Principle of Synchronicity

Earlier that day in Memphis, I had lunch with some old friends. During lunch, they discussed a cassette tape that one of the women had brought to give to another. She was telling everyone how wonderful it was. I felt drawn to the information it contained and surprised everyone, including myself, when I asked to borrow the tape for myself. I did not know why I wanted it, but I convinced her to loan it to me. I now know the Universe is always putting things in our paths, having people say something or give us something at the right time. It may be a book or a tape that comes into your hands at a time you need it most. This is called the Principle of Synchronicity.

As I returned to my motel later that day, I had forgotten about the tape, so I was planning to watch TV. As synchronicity would have it, the TV did not work, and I felt it unwise to leave the room because of the dangerous area of the city in which I had found myself. A long afternoon stretched ahead before my evening meeting. Out of desperation, I thought of the tape. I rummaged around until I found it, then popped it into my traveling tape recorder, leaned back in my chair and began to listen.

The speaker had a foreign accent, which I found very difficult to understand. He identified himself as a medical doctor, an endocrinologist. I thought to myself, "Oh, brother. I can hardly understand him, and he is talking about things I do not know anything about. This isn't working for me."

Nevertheless, destitute in my misery, I continued to listen. Just as some of you reading this book may not relate to my experience so far, I promise you that, if you will stick with it, there may be something for you. The man was speaking in a monotone voice, certainly not the dramatic highs and lows of the type of preaching I did, nor the type of speaking I was used to hearing. Without the emotional stimulus that typically comes from variations in vocal tone, I was getting very bored.

Halfway through the tape, with my head bobbing, dozing semi-conscious in and out, this heavily accented voice suddenly said, "What we believed to be empty space in the human cell, through old Newtonian physics, is actually, in the new quantum physics, a teeming Field of All Possibilities. When we realize that our true self is one of pure potentiality, we can then align ourselves with the power that manifests everything in the Universe." (Chopra 1993) (Original 1988 tape series no longer available)

Hit By Lightning!

I bolted up out of my trance-like semi-consciousness as though hit by lightning. I felt electrified throughout every cell of my body. Every tiny particle of myself was teeming and tingling with creative potential; trembling in a Field that felt like musical notes, dancing together in unlimited harmonies and songs full of the life force. This life force exuded happiness, good health, energy, enthusiasm for life, fulfilling relationships, creative and secure financial freedom, along with emotional and psychological stability. This life force brought to me a complete sense of well-being, happiness, and joy. Most importantly, it brought peace of mind through the awareness of an abundance exponentially greater than I had ever experienced. My whole being seemed to be screaming, "Everything is possible. Everything is potential. The mystery is finished." I immediately had a cellular knowing that what religion refers to as "spirit" is actually our human potential.

During this experience I remembered a poem that I had seen on the wall of a church we were using for our meetings in Denver. It was a poem written by English poet Christopher Logue:

Come to the edge.
We can't. We are afraid.
Come to the edge.
We can't. We will fall.
Come to the edge.
And they came.
And he pushed them.
And they flew.

The whole of Creation was standing on its tiptoes, beckoning for me to come forth. It was beckoning me to step into THE EVERYTHING that lives, moves, and has its being in a moment-by-moment, glorious demonstration of perfect happiness, deep well-being, peace, and joyous celebration. It was an invitation to be a part of THE EVERYTHING that has its being in full knowledge of its purpose and intention for being alive. How exciting – the possibility of being in harmony and working together with everything else in a non-hierarchical system of shared information and energy. One part of me felt I would jump to my absolute ruin. However, another part was so excited that I could not wait to fly into the field of endless possibility.

Do you remember the void, the vast emptiness that I saw? The man on the tape was telling me that *nothing* is the place of *everything*, in its purest form. *No-thingness* is unlimited potential – the birthplace, the womb of our consciousness. Dr. Deepak Chopra was the voice on the tape in that motel room in Memphis.

Today, I experience God as energy, intelligent energy, a non-local, non-material intelligent energy interacting with itself in all dimensions, in all places, at all times. As Meister Eckhart reminds us, "The *idea* of God can become the final obstacle to God." Therefore, an experience of God is always more enlightening than an idea of God.

A Sacred Sound Within Me

I began to hear a sacred sound developing within me. The sound became a thought and I knew it was a first great thought of this cycle of enlightenment. It was divine thought thinking through me, as me. I knew that I had now become available so that the Universe could flow freely through me and bring a new energy and light to the planet. I recalled something a visionary had told me many years before: that I had incarnated as part of a Family of Lightworkers *"to set the Ordinances of Heaven into the Earth."* I now understood what this meant.

I saw this possibility in a new way, in a new light. Verses from Genesis flowed through my mind with a new understanding: "...And the earth was without form and void; and darkness was upon the face of the deep [...] and God vibrated (moved) across the face of the deep and said, 'Let there be light,' and there was light."

Michael Talbot, referencing David Bohm in *Holographic Universe* (1992) Void does not mean space that is empty – it is full – a plenum. A plenum as opposed to a vacuum is the ground for the existence of everything, including ourselves. We find that every cubic centimeter of empty space contains more energy than the total energy of all matter in the universe. (51) When the silence of the void is activated, it begins to vibrate and hum, manifesting as primordial sound. First, there is sound, then the thought, followed by the pouring forth of light: thus, the thought form is filled with light. This thought form created by the sound is a source of enlightenment, for it reveals Truth and brings an aspect of reality to the consciousness of the observer. This light is the teeming Field of all Possibilities. As I sat in the motel in Memphis, the light filled the room and permeated every cell of my body.

Dr. Guiliana Conforto in *Man's Cosmic Game* (1999) says, "Every cell pulsates, absorbs, reflects and interacts with the acoustic oscillations of the medium." This was my very real experience. Some people call this an *Epiphany*. The Buddhists call it a moment of enlightenment. I have heard it said that an epiphany is *when the gods show up*. To me, an epiphany is a moment of realization and revelation that can change everything. It is the ending of something and the beginning something else. It is a moment of being out of time and space, of being one with all things, cut loose from the past and future. I call it my SACRED PAUSE. The Bible calls it "thirty minutes of Silence in Heaven" *(Revelation 8:1)*. It is the point where the pendulum pauses for a nanosecond before reversing its swing. In the *Biology of Transcendence* by Joseph Pearce Chilton, Carlos Castaneda's metaphor of a "cubic centimeter of chance" (15) describes a nanosecond where a new opportunity opens and closes, almost like a single pulse. We must fall through at the instant of its opening, or we will miss the opportunity.

I do not know how long my Sacred Pause lasted, but I believe that time stood still at that moment. I was out of time – out of the time of the past and not yet in the time of the future. I was in THE FIELD described by the poet Rumi in the 13th century when he wrote, "Out beyond ideas of wrongdoing and right doing there is a field. I will meet you there." I remembered Jesus had talked about the field, saying that in the field there was a pearl of great price. I was in this Field, a teeming Field of All Possibilities. In quantum physics, this Field is a living void, pulsating in endless rhythms of creation and destruction. The Field is where virtual particles spontaneously come into being out of the void and vanish again into the void without any other interacting particle being present. Dr. Deepak Chopra calls this *The Gap*, the place between thoughts, the place where all is possible.

I Had To Get Real

After that glorious experience in the motel room in Memphis, I knew I had to rethink my life and become completely honest with myself. I had to get *real*.

We have to be *real* when we stand in the light. I could see the authentic me. I could feel the authentic me. I stood there in the light. I was pure, virtuous, innocent, and eager. I wanted to literally remember the authentic me. I wanted to begin the path of *undoing* all of the things that had created the false me, the miserable me, my pseudo-self, what I understand now to be the ego.

In the light of all possibilities, I could see a path laid out before me. I instinctively knew that this path led to realms of enlightenment, revelation, and wisdom that would move me to my next work in this earthwalk. I would venture into Realms containing information that could not have been told to me before and be given Information that was for TODAY, information needed for THIS MOMENT. I could not have handled it before. I was not ready for it before. I had to be brought to my Sacred Pause before I would be willing to hear what my spiritual guides were going to teach me.

I knew in my bones that this path led to places where few had traveled before and was filled with crosses and graves, crosses on which the brave ones were crucified, their lives ridiculed, their work sabotaged, and their careers destroyed. Brave men like Nikola Tesla and Raymond Rife. I did not know their names at that moment, but I learned them later as I journeyed down the path. I instinctively knew that I was about to undergo a dramatic revealing of myself – my pseudo-self and my authentic self.

Angry at God

I dared to let the first layer unfold. I was eager to get started. I wanted to know everything. I was ready to release all of the layers of information and misinformation that had formerly validated my beliefs. I began to realize that I was angry, very, very angry. A process of enlightenment often begins with confronting anger. I was angry with myself and I was angry with God. I felt God had called me to preach at sixteen years old and I blamed *God* for taking me away from a normal teen-age life, and putting on my innocent shoulders the awesome responsibility to see that the whole world was saved. I believed God was telling me, through the Bible to "Go ye into all the world, and preach the gospel to the whole creation." (Mark 16:15) And, "For this is good and acceptable in the sight of God our Saviour; Who will have all men to be saved, and to come unto the knowledge of the truth" (1 Tim. 2:3-4).

I was taught that the World would go to a burning, tormenting Hell if I did not preach to it. I was sure that God wanted me to do my part in helping everyone be *saved* and make it to *The Rapture* before the great tribulations begin.

In retrospect, I realized that I was angry because I thought that God had put such a terrible responsibility upon me. I was angry that I had to live by faith, never having a secure paycheck or retirement program, never knowing how much money was going to come in to cover all the expenses. Many times, I felt that I had not aligned myself to my soul's purpose. I married and had a daughter, only to realize quickly that this marriage was not going to work out, and I divorced. Now I was a divorced, non-denominational preacher trying to earn a living by preaching a message about love, healing, and being Sons of God. I was angry with God for letting all of this happen to me. I felt victimized. As a teenager, I had felt validated by God. Now I realized that I felt invalidated by God, fearful, and alone.

In my moment of enlightenment, standing in The Gap – my Sacred Pause, and looking at my real Self, I began to unplug my energy from all the preconceived ideas and teachings about the God of organized religion. I began to trust my real Self who had never been influenced by anything I was taught by my parents, by schools, by society, by religion – that part of me that is pure, untouched, and un-penetrated by the systems of the world, that virgin part of me. I began to trust that part of me that is One with Source, that has always been One with Source.

Unplugging my energy reminded me of my experience as a young man, watching my mother who worked as a telephone switchboard operator for Southwestern Bell. I used to watch her pull out lines and plug in new lines as she worked at the switchboard. I saw myself as one of those great big switchboards with all the lines plugged into sockets. I just began pulling out my old beliefs. I became unplugged from many of the belief systems of my youth. In my mind, I watched as my pseudo self began to melt into my real self. Then my real self walked up to the edge of the light I saw in my Sacred Pause.

Again, remembering the poem by Christopher Logue that had influenced me at the beginning of this journey, I feel it is worth repeating for those of you who may be standing at the edge in your lives, as I was at that moment:

> *Come to the edge.*
> *We can't. We are afraid.*
> *Come to the edge.*
> *We can't. We will fall.*
> *Come to the edge.*
> *And they came.*
> *And he pushed them.*
> *And they flew.*

Then, at the edge, I, David Hulse, prayed as David in the Bible prayed: "Oh God make me like you, who sees darkness and light as the same." (Psalms. 139) Again, David said, "God has made darkness His secret place, His pavilion." (Psalms 18.11) Then a voice at my shoulder said, "My son, there are no accidents. It is no accident that YOU are named David." I took one step into my own nothingness and I dove into the darkness.

A Course In Miracles

Soon after this experience, I was introduced to the ministry of Marianne Williamson who taught A Course In Miracles (The Course). The Course is a spiritual psychological system that shifts us from fear-based to love-based perceptions of the world and ourselves. It presents a different idea about many fear-based doctrines of the Bible and offers a fresh approach to interpreting the Bible. From The Course I understood that I was not a dirty sinner who constantly needed saving. Rather, God had always loved me. God had never seen me as a sinner, but always as a perfect spiritual idea within the Divine Mind, complete, lacking nothing. That was revolutionary. It changed everything.. This later became part of the basic premise of my development of the SomaEnergetics teachings, which I explore in detail later in this book.

A Course in Miracles said that "I was God's beloved child filled with love, light, innocence, curiosity, and playfulness." (Schucman 2007) God had given me the opportunity to experience life by making choices. I was given the opportunity to finish what God had started in creating me. Just as we as parents take our children to certain points in their lives, and then turn them loose to experience life for themselves, so too God turns us loose to experience life. It seems that God has *seeded* the earth with holograms of Himself. The seeds wait to be activated into life by certain triggers or key frequencies. We incarnate with a certain amount of information and knowledge, and then we make daily choices in life that can lead us to finding the yellow roses of our lives. I believe we have Divine seeds (codes) within us at this very moment that can be activated by the use of certain missing sounds and frequencies.

A Course in Miracles was a very attractive bridge I wanted to walk across to greater and deeper realms of understanding. It was a bridge that beckoned to my soul's longing and made my spirit sing and dance. I discovered later that when our insides begin to sing and dance, it is called *resonance*. I was resonating with information from the outside of me that was agreeing with information on the inside of me – information I brought into this life that was stored in my bones. Many say that this inner knowing is Information that is vibrationally imprinted on the iron in our red blood cells. All the cells of my body were saying, *yes, yes, yes!*

As I meditated about healing, I began to realize that healing does not come from some power outside of us or some God in the sky. I realized that all of the healings I had witnessed in my ministry actually came from inside the people being healed when they connected to their inherent inner faith. It was their faith (intent) that allowed higher consciousness to reconnect with their authentic self as many great teachers have said, "by thy faith thou art healed."

God does not choose to heal one person, and choose not to heal someone else. The ability to heal is within each and every person. Those who have been living at the survival level feel an attraction to be at a higher level of consciousness. The degree to which each is able to activate and avail themselves of this power determines the extent to which a person experiences healing. Any facilitator who works in the healing arts is merely one who provides a safe place of non-judgment and unconditional love so people can heal themselves. Healing is remembering and reconnecting with our authentic, perfect Self – a self that exists beyond all time.

CHAPTER TWO - THE DARKNESS

Light has need of darkness -- otherwise how could it appear as light?
Carl Jung

THERE ARE TREASURES IN THE DARKNESS. Isaiah 45:3

THE DARKNESS AND LIGHT ARE BOTH ALIKE TO THEE. Psalms 139:12

In my Western mind, I had thought of nothing as *no-thing*. Yet, to the Eastern mind, *nothing* is where *everything* is. My fundamentalist background taught that the devil and demons were in the darkness. They were there hiding and they were trying to trick me in order to get my soul. To the Eastern mind, darkness is the source of the light — darkness is where the mystery of God is. The mystery of God is hidden information, information that has been kept from the masses. When I dove into my darkness, I was not plunged to my utter ruin, as I had feared. I entered into a new adventure that promised to explain the mystery of God in my own life. I was in new, unbounded and uncharted territory. All things were becoming new.

I was so tired of being told I would "understand it better in the "By and By," as the old gospel hymn states. Preachers have preached for generations that when we get to Heaven, we will "finally understand everything." They never had answers for any of life's mysteries right now. All of my WHY questions were largely unanswered. I wanted answers now. I wanted understanding now. I believed that deep call within me for this understanding was what created the circumstances that brought me to my Sacred Pause moment. Coming to the Sacred Pause moment allowed me to learn that the end of something is always the beginning of something else. Coming to the end of something occurs when something new wants to be born. Coming to the end of this 3rd time/space continuum, I believe many are experiencing their last incarnation, therefore making birth and death a simultaneous event. We begin a new circle of learning, a new level of experience and understanding – a new paradigm.

Instead of going off the edge of that cliff to my utter ruin, I flew into the Field of All Possibilities. In Matthew 13:14, the author states, "The Kingdom of God is like unto a treasure hid in a field, that when a man finds it, he is so filled with joy, he sells all that he has in order to buy the field." I had found the Field. I began to "sell all that I had" by getting rid of many of the beliefs that had their source outside of myself, as they no longer aligned with my new inner understandings. It took all the faith and energy I had at that moment to make these changes; yet instinctively, I knew that I could investigate anything in this new realm, fearlessly and excitedly. I felt totally free to begin to pursue new ideas, new thoughts, to begin to satisfy the longings of my heart. I felt very free to look into anything, or everything, with no fear of being wrong, no fear of being outcast, and no fear of being lost.

I could not run fast enough to start intensively studying *A Course in Miracles*. If you put *A Course in Miracles* into any search engine on the Internet, you'll find answers to all of the questions you might have about The Course. For two years, I studied The Course, and I began to teach it at many of my conferences. I was no longer afraid of investigating what The Course was saying. I discovered that almost everything it taught was already in the Bible and that I was already familiar with much of the terminology used in The Course.

Take Another Look

As I studied, I began to see things differently, moving from a fear-based philosophy to a love-based perception of what the Bible said. I took another look at some of my traditional ideas and concepts about such topics as heaven, hell, sin, the devil, and judgment. I began to release myself from the fear-based manipulating and controlling rules and regulations developed by those who established the religious systems here on Earth. Eventually I wrote a book about my findings titled *Take Another Look: A Scriptural Review of Traditional Christian Doctrines* (1999)[1].

As I expanded my horizons by studying *A Course In Miracles*, I could feel the warm holy breath of Spirit melting the ice of my beliefs that lay frozen and locked within me and releasing the free flow of God's love and energy in my life. One of my favorite passages is by Christopher Fry, from his play entitled "A Sleep of Prisoners (1951)"

> The human heart can go the lengths of God
> Dark and cold we may be, but this
> Is no winter now. The frozen misery
> Of century's breaks, cracks, begins to move;
> The thunder is the thunder of the floes,
> The thaw, the flood, the upstart spring.
> Thank God our time is now when wrong
> Comes up to face us everywhere,
> Never to leave us till we take
> The longest stride of soul men ever took.
> Affairs are now soul size.
> The enterprise is exploration into God.
> Where are you waiting for?
> It takes so many thousand years to wake
> But will you wake, for pity's sake?

Good and Very Good

A Course in Miracles is a wonderful bridge that people who wish to make a transition in perception can journey across in their search for Truth. I loved every word, every idea, and every new way of looking at the former beliefs that were not

---

[1] This book is available on my website, www.lightwithin.com.

working for me anymore. I began to experience the Truth as wondrous rivers of living water flowing through me, energizing me, and setting me free from the dangerous and manipulating ideas of organized religion that had caused me pain and suffering for so long.

Over the next weeks, months, and years, my icebergs of guilt and fear just melted away in the rich warm waters of God's love and God's acceptance of me. I came to feel as though God could actually be proud of me. I felt I was really growing up and becoming more responsible, feeling more and more of my own divinity. I felt more relaxed, more rested.

I floated in the waters. I let the waters take me along in the flow of life. I got rid of evaluative labels such as "right and wrong," and "good and bad." Those were just labels of my own making. Since I was the one putting the labels on things, I could be the one to change them. I could rename something I had called "bad," and call it "good," living what Shakespeare had expressed so succinctly in the play *Hamlet*: "there is nothing either good or bad, but thinking makes it so. (Act II, Scene 2)" I learned that God only has two standards of judgment: good and very good. I decided that everything in my life was now good or very good.

A Course in Miracles and the Unified Field

My experience in Memphis also quickened my interest in exploring the evolving world of quantum physics. Dr. Deepak Chopra used a considerable amount of information from the realm of physics to explain some of the fundamental spiritual principles he was discussing. Having no academic background in physics, I found myself wanting to know more about it. In *The Holographic Universe* (1992), by Michael Talbot I read about the fascinating world of subatomic particles. The subatomic level is filled with particles and waves, atoms, photons, nucleons, quarks, and gluons. I read about electromagnetic fields that can travel through space in the form of radio waves, light waves, and other kinds of electromagnetic radiation.

Talbot's book discusses the hologram. The hologram appears to go beyond the quantum physics realm of probabilities to explore an implicit order that seems to prevail throughout the Cosmos at a deeper, non-manifest level. Each part of a hologram contains the whole. If any part of a hologram is available, the entire image can be reconstructed.

The example of the hologram proved to me that God is in everything. Many physicists today, including David Bohm the forerunner in this field of study who calls his theory Holomovement, believe that the real world is structured according to holographic principles. This means that the whole is enfolded in each of its parts. The hologram theory links quantum physics and Einstein's relativity theory. Bohm believes that to be able to fully understand this implicit order, it is necessary to regard consciousness as an essential feature of the *Holomovement*. Bohm sees "mind and matter as being interdependent and correlated...mutually enfolding projections of a higher reality which is neither matter nor consciousness (Capra,1975:320)."

After this heady foray into quantum mechanics and the contemporary Holomovement, I thought to myself that my definition of God is not so far-out. God as a non-local, non-material, intelligent energy interacting with itself thoroughly aligns with contemporary theoretical physics. Nevertheless, I puzzled over how energy works in relationship with itself. It has to have the ability to simultaneously raise and lower its frequency, resulting in a spectrum of vibration reaching all the way from the lower x-rays to the higher gamma rays.

Everything is Relationship!

Part of my answer to this was that everything is relationship. No one, no thing is alone and apart. Everything is connected. Everyone is a part of everyone else, and everything is a part of everything else in the Unified Field. In quantum physics, unified field theory is an attempt to unify all the fundamental forces and the interactions between elementary particles into a single theoretical framework. As in physics, so too in everyday life. We cannot continue to be passive observers, just watching the game of life, or sitting in a pew awaiting our spoon feeding. We are called by spirit and can become active in our roles as co-creative partners with the energy.

According to Dr. Fred Wolf, who is also known as Dr. Quantum, when you are observing an object, on some level the object is observing you. The observer and the observed are one. (Wolf 2000). While considering this, I looked at the glass of water sitting on my desk. I observed it. Was the glass of water also observing me? The glass of water was half empty. On the other hand, was it half full? I guess my observation of the glass of water would determine this. The glass of water looked to me for its definition. Fascinating. I decided the glass was half-full.

Second Great Spiritual Experience –
The Life Review Vision

One morning, as I floated on the waters of my meditation, I had an Open Vision. An Open Vision has substance and is filled with sounds and sights. I was in meditation, but I was awake and aware. I saw three Beings of Light, a trio of Entities, sitting at a table. The Beings were non-corporal, pulsing forms of love and acceptance. While they did not speak in a human way, saying words or communicating in sentences, I still knew what they were thinking and saying to me, mind to mind. I felt very open and exposed to them, and had absolutely no fear or trepidation.

During this experience, I noticed that they were not separate in any way from me. I was part of them and they were part of me. It is hard to explain this, but I just knew that we were all one great big entity together. They reviewed my previous lives, and then they began to let me view the incarnation I am in now. They said to me that a new energy was coming to earth from a higher dimension of life. They said that because this is a free will planet, not enough souls had yet achieved a level of consciousness to be able to stabilize this new energy. It would, therefore, take enough souls to incarnate now and live, in one lifetime, what would be the equivalent of many lifetimes. They had asked for those who would choose to incarnate and live this experience. I had volunteered to be one of these souls.

Let me tell you, in one nanosecond I saw that planet Earth is one hot piece of real estate in God's multiple-listing directory of the Universe. It is not because Earth is in the center of things. The sun does not go around the Earth; the earth rotates around the sun, and even our solar system is not in the center of things. We are stuck out here at the edge of the Milky Way Galaxy, far away from almost everything, out here in the boon docks. When the Hubble telescope takes pictures one way, it looks into the Milky Way Galaxy. When it takes pictures looking the opposite way, it looks out into NOTHING! (Remember, the vast realm of no-thing holds the potential for everything.)

A New Energy is Coming

My vision continued with the knowing that a new energy is coming on the Earth now. Things are speeding up. Time is becoming more relative than it ever has been. The electromagnetic fields of the Earth are changing, old things are passing away, and everything is becoming new. Nothing can be hidden anymore. No more secrets – no more powers outside ourselves manipulating and controlling us. This new energy needs to be stabilized and grounded. Who will ground the energy? Where are the Lightworkers? I thought that maybe the Earth, too, is reaching its own Sacred Pause experience.

I began to realize that the collective consciousness of Earth had to be raised to a level that could stabilize the new energy that is coming in now. I saw that this energy of a higher frequency had come to the planet before, could not be stabilized, and Earth had been destroyed in a cycle that has occurred repeatedly. I saw that if there were enough souls who would volunteer to help stabilize the higher energies, we could make it this time and advance to the next order of things for our planet. We have a long, long way to go, and not a lot of time available to do it. We have had the opportunity to evolve before, but our personal integrity and global moralities never gained enough power to master the technologies necessary for advancement and the technologies destroyed us.

I saw that I had agreed to be one of the souls who would help our planet to transition this time. I saw that I had given the "Board of Entities" a resounding YES, telling them that I wanted to be a part of this group. I said, "Give me all you've got to get me ready."

I've crowded many lifetimes of experience into my life this time to be prepared to hold this new energy for myself, and then be able to teach others to hold it. I saw all the times in my life where I had held the energy for a while, and then let it go. Again and again, I held it for a while, and let it go. I saw that now it is time for me to hold the energy and stay in the new vibration.

I now know that I have been a part of all decisions that contoured my present life situations. I have approved every decision concerning my incarnation, and I have confirmed every decision affecting every part of my life since I have been here. I saw the times I had denied responsibility for what had happened in my life. I had blamed God for the things I had called "bad." I had made God my scapegoat. I decided to release God from any responsibility. No one else had caused my situations. I and I alone have chosen and validated everything for myself. I take complete responsibility.

A Free Will Planet

What makes Earth such an important place is the Universal Christ Consciousness manifested on this planet in the person of Jesus. (Finding out who Jesus really is can be another fascinating journey.) The second reason Earth is such an important place is because it is a place where the free will of the human being is supreme. There are other types of planetary experiences in the vast Universe where our solar system dwells. There are other planets where life is more structured and less volatile. However, on a free will planet, God has no preferences. Life is an adventure on a free will planet. The Creator can only experience adventurous life in the Creation when that Creation has the power to make choices. In addition, the love experienced in a free will zone is much deeper and much more satisfying than it is in a preplanned and predestined environment.

This satisfaction emerges from the fact that everyone in a free will zone creates everything that happens in that place. Everyone in a free will zone has to choose everything for his or her life. *Even not choosing* is making a choice. We have created "evil" so we can know what "good" is. Remember Shakespeare wrote, "There is nothing either good or bad, but *thinking* makes it so."

God sees everything that happens in a free will zone as pure adventure. Just think about it. God sees me as an adventure in human living. God sees you as an adventure in human living. God is experiencing the adventures of the alcoholic, the prostitute, the heterosexual, the homosexual, the clerk at McDonalds, the CEO of a huge corporation, the liberal, the conservative, the black, the Muslim, the woman, the man. The human race here on Earth is God's adventure in the experience of itself. Remember my new definition of God: namely, that *God is a non-local, non-material intelligence that interacts with itself.* God is in us, and we are part of God, something that we can experience in interaction with each other. If you do not think this is fair, then the next time you incarnate, just tell the "Board of Entities" that you want to go to a controlled, predetermined planet. Personally, I love being an Adventure. My sense of curiosity and desire for excitement make this planet extremely interesting. Remember I am a Sagittarius.

Consider, for a moment, that nothing is good or bad of itself. Nothing is right or wrong. Everything is an experience. We are the ones who are the label maker, choosing to print the words "good" or "bad." Remember this Truth, let it resonate through you, and your life will be transformed. I keep saying it repeatedly because such Truths are the basis of our perception. We can just release all regrets, all judgments, and all feelings of failure. We can embrace everything that has ever happened in our lives– the good times, the bad times, the uptimes, the downtimes – all are the riches of our adventure as human beings and make Source rich by experiencing itself as us. All things work together for the highest good – literally everyone and everything on the planet. We cannot separate ourselves from the others who live here, no matter where they live or what they do. We are all one planet. We are all one Creation. We are all Co-Creators.

The person who started me on this journey, Dr. Deepak Chopra, says in his audio series *Higher Self* (1993), "Your individual role in life is to manifest the things you desire in life." Our role is not to try to see how we can get someone else to manifest what is in our heart-of-hearts for us, nor to wait until we die, go to Heaven, and then receive our desires. Dr. Chopra continues, "Once you increasingly manifest what you want, your sense of being a creator steadily enlarges until you eventually realize that everything is available to you. This is a state of total freedom." Dr. Chopra calls this UNITY CONSCIOUSNESS. I call it getting real and knowing who you are. You are in charge of your life. If we remember just this one thing, our lives will be forever altered and changed: we have the power to become whatever we want to be. We can do whatever we desire to do. The book and DVD entitled *The Secret* point clearly to this principle. (Byrne 2006)

The 144,000

I've often wondered if all the souls who made this same choice – to hold the new energy and incarnate now – are the 144,000 talked about in the *Book of Revelation* in the *Bible*. Accordingly, these 144,000 sing a new song, and no man could learn that song but the 144,000 who were redeemed from the Earth. I do not believe that 144,000 is a literal number of people. Using Pythagorean numerical reduction, 144,000 becomes a nine. (1+4+4 equals 9). Nine is the spiritual number of completion. Once we realize that we are without fault, we can learn this song, The song, I believe is composed of certain notes that have very specific frequencies. When we know who we are as complete and whole beings, lacking nothing, then, and only then, may we become God's song on Earth.

I saw that I had decided that a free will planet would give me the most opportunity to experience all that I could be. I saw that these decisions were then encoded in my DNA and stored in my bones. I chose my parents. I chose those certain genetic codes through my parents that determined my height, my appearance (my nose is not God's nose – it's exactly like my father's) the color of my eyes, my talents and my gifts. I came into life knowing how to play the piano. I never took piano lessons; I could just go to the piano and play and sing. That was all part of the preparation for leading me to sing the New Song, and I came ready to accompany myself on the piano.

I had learned that life is a gift, but one's journey is about choices. I had chosen to be a preacher. I had chosen to get married. I had chosen to have a daughter. I had chosen every step of my way. I began to have such peace with myself. I could feel the anger melting away as I began to remember the spirit of my mission while being present in my body. I had chosen to come. I was finally awake to the Divine Plan organizing my life; all things that had happened to me were in my sacred Contract. I was not a victim.

Remember this Truth: *there are no mistakes*. There are no errors. We have never been wrong. We have never done what we should not do. Everything is part of the process. When we realize that we chose to come here, that we have a specific reason for being here, and when we find out what it is and begin doing it, we see how everything that has ever happened to us was all part of the process. We begin to be connected in harmony with all things and all people.

Dear reader, stay with me now. The path is full of surprises, twists, and turns. Adventure lies around each corner. Do not be afraid to take another look. Becoming a part of the critical mass, the figurative 144,000 souls, prepares us to learn the song using the ancient frequencies of sound. Could using these ancient frequencies being restored to us at this time, be a catalyst for learning the new song?

The Frequency to Repair DNA

At this point in my life, someone gave me an article about Dr. Leonard G. Horowitz's book *Healing Codes for the Biological Apocalypse* (1999). This article talked about a mystic revelation that was received by Dr. Joseph Puleo. Dr. Puleo found codes in the *Bible* that revealed a series of six electro-magnetic sound frequencies that correspond to the six missing tones of the ancient Solfeggio. The article also spoke of one of these tones, the MI frequency which occurs at 528 hertz, and how this frequency is currently being used by genetic biochemists to repair broken DNA.

NOW I WAS EXCITED. There it was - a frequency to work with and repair DNA. I was ecstatic. When I started on this path, I had no idea I would discover such an important and significant piece of information as this seemed to be. Was this true that DNA is not set in stone, as I once thought? Can

DNA sequencing be altered? The implication is that by using a specific frequency, hereditary weaknesses and strengths can be altered by returning them to homeostasis or balance. On a personal level, that would mean I did not have to follow my father through the experience of heart trouble at the age of 61.

Could it be that everything, including our DNA, can be altered, completely changed, by the right intention and frequency? A tone can change cellular structures and patterns. The right vibrations can enter a diseased cell and that cell can be completely returned to normal. All we need to do is sound the right tone. Cymatics, the science of vibration and form is empirical proof that sound alters matter. A more detailed discussion of Cymatics comes later in the book.

Researchers such as Royal Raymond Rife[1] discovered frequencies that destroy disease-causing viruses and bacteria. He was right. His life work was discredited, even endangered, at the time; however, because it was such a threat to traditional western medicine. It is good to see that today's science is beginning to vindicate him and that his research was not in vain [see *The End of All Disease*, by R. E. Payne (2003)].

Dr. Candace Pert, Ph.D. pharmacologist, says in *Molecules of Emotion* (1999) that receptors on the cell membrane are perpetually scanning their immediate environment for the right dancing ligand to turn them on. Dr. Pert asserts that this binding is analogous to "two voices striking the same note and producing a vibration that rings a doorbell to open the cell doorway." (24) To me it seems logical that this 528 Hz tone could also be a dancing key much in the same way a ligand is, holding the potential to opening the doorway to the cell and reaching the water molecules that make up our DNA.

---

[1] The following websites carry more information about Rife: www.rense.com/general31/rife.htm or www.amazon.com

Dr. Lee Lorenzen, PhD is using the 528 Hertz frequency to create clustered water. His discussion in *Healing Codes for the Biological Apocalypse* (Horowitz 1999) emphasizes the importance of sacred geometry in the optimal functioning of healthy DNA; in particular, six-sided hexagonal structured water molecules are said to "form the supportive matrix of healthy DNA (180)." He goes on to suggest that the depletion of this matrix is a fundamental process "underlying aging [that] negatively affects virtually every physiological function. (180)

Remember, 528 Hz is one of the six frequencies of the Solfeggio. It is a musical tone – and unlike chemicals or drugs, it has no unhealthy side effects or any chance of dependency. What a wondrous way to assist in the healing process. Play music. Sound the right tone.

Another Epiphany: I thought to myself, "Well, then, I'll just go to my piano and sound the "Mi" note, and I'll fix everything that is wrong with me." After all, we all know the following about the 12-tone temperament: "Do, a deer, a female deer, Re, a drop of golden Sun, Mi, a name I call myself, Fa, a long, long way to run (*Sound of Music*. (1965)." I could see Julie Andrews running up over the top of the mountain, with the goats and the sheep, singing Do, Re, Mi, Fa, Sol, La, Ti, Do. So, to my piano I did run. Alas, I discovered that the C note on my piano was only 512 hertz and NOT 528 hertz.

CHAPTER THREE – JUST INTONATION & 12-TONE EQUAL TEMPERAMENT

My next stop along the process was my piano tuner's home. My question to him was, "How in the world do you tune my piano?" His response was, "With an A-440." I said, "440 hertz?" He said yes. I asked, "How did the Mi note get from 528 hertz to 512 hertz?" He said, "Because of 12-Tone Temperament. The old Mi note was tuned in a different temperament, probably Just Intonation." I had played the piano all of my life and never once thought about HOW my piano was tuned. Why were there different tunings of instruments? Was it always this way? Why was there more than one temperament?

After that discussion, I felt compelled to surf the Internet, I did a search using the keyword "temperament." Wikipedia provided the following: "In musical tuning, a *temperament* is a system of tuning which slightly compromises the pure intervals of just intonation in order to meet other requirements of the system." (http://en.wikipedia.org/wiki/Musical_temperament) A lot of the information I found is beyond the scope of this book. But, at its essence, music is mathematics – intervals, integers, fractions, and ratios. And music is sound. Sound is vibration, with the frequencies measured in hertz. Music has pitch, partials, majors, minors, thirds, fifths, sixths, sevenths, and ninths. There are also several different methods of tuning: Mean Tone Temperament, Just Intonation, Pythagorean tuning, and 12-Tone (or Equal) Temperament.

Today, most Western musical compositions and instruments, including pianos and organs, are tuned according to 12-Tone Equal Temperament. From an article on the Internet that discusses the differences between Just Intonation and 12-Tone Equal Temperament, Kyle Gann, a contemporary Composer, musicologist, writer, and educator says:

> [...]12-tone equal temperament chords have a kind of active buzz to them, a level of harmonic excitement and intensity. By contrast, just-intonation chords are much calmer and more passive; you literally have to slow down to listen to them. As Terry Riley says, 'Western music is fast because it's not in tune.' Most cultures use music for meditation. Our culture may be the only one that does not. With 12-tone equal Temperament tuning, we can't (1997). (Gann 2008)

Kyle Gann continues by retelling what his teacher, Ben Johnston told him.

> Johnston believed that our tuning system is responsible for much of our cultural psychology, the fact that we are so geared toward progress, action, and violence and so little attuned to introspection, contentment and bliss. A 12-Tone Equal Temperament "diet" could be described as the musical equivalent to eating a lot of red meat and processed sugars and watching violent action movies. The music does not turn your attention inward. It makes you want to go out and work off your nervous energy on something...or someone.

Kyle Gann states that composing and listening to music tuned in Just Intonation creates tranquil, purely consonant harmony. Listening to 12-Tone Equal Temperament creates a kind of aural caffeine, an overly busy and very nervous experience. Just Intonation music sensitizes one to a myriad of colors while 12-Tone Equal Temperament is like seeing everything click back to black and white.

The original Christian Church Fathers also recognized that certain tones fostered the relationship between human beings, as the Creation and God, as the Creator. This relationship is exemplified in the relationship between sound and form.

The earliest church music was Plain Chant, of which the Gregorian chant is best known. Some of these hymns and chants were based on the original Solfeggio scale of Ut, Re, Mi, Fa, Sol and La. At this point in my journey there was another Sacred Pause: is the MI note in the original chants, based on the original Solfeggio scale, the Mi that was the 528 Hz?

The primary characteristic of a chant is simplicity. A chant consists of a single melodic tone, which commonly travels up or down gradually, one-step at a time. As the tones step up, human consciousness rises into higher dimensions of thought and awareness and can more easily be exposed to the God Self. According to Dr. Leonard Horowitz in *Healing Codes for the Biological Apocalypse.* (1999) Professor Willi Apel of Indiana University conducted research into the history of the Ut note. His inquiry determined that these original Gregorian chants were tampered with and the Ut note was dropped. Ut was artificially replaced by the Do note, and the 7th note Si was added. Si was later changed to Ti to avoid confusion with Sol. This completely changed the chants and, not unexpectedly, began to dull the minds of the masses who used them. The changed chants effectively severed humanity from the God Self, separating human from the divine.

Here was the missing piece in my research, historical record of when the Ut note was dropped and the Si note added. Is it possible that the medieval Christian Church did not want their people to get in touch with the God Self? This would give the individual their God power. The Church wanted to be the power and to tell people what to do. They altered the original notes. They dropped the Ut and added the Ti.

In the Dark Ages, old paradigms dictated that information was to be kept from the masses. Only professionals could know the *secrets*. There were well-established lineages of secret-keepers for this purpose. This began the separation that was mirrored across the spiritual, temporal, and human realms — God from humans, church from state, and humans from other humans. Religions were developed that separated human beings and those religions continue to cause havoc on our earth today.

When Dr. Joseph Puleo, naturopathic physician, and co-author of *Healing Codes for the Biological Apocalypse* (1999) was researching the tones, he "was directed to a monsignor at a university in Spokane, WA who headed the Medieval Department. Dr. Puleo asked the Monsignor, 'Can you decipher Medieval Latin?' The Monsignor said emphatically, 'Absolutely.' Dr. Puleo asked, 'And you know the musical scale and everything?' The Monsignor said, 'Absolutely.' Dr. Puleo said, 'Well then, could you tell me what UT – QUEANT LAXIS means?' The Monsignor quipped, 'It's none of your business,' and he hung up." (Horowitz 71) That has been the position of most of the governing hierarchies of the earth. It is none of our business? I am telling you, my friends, it definitely is OUR BUSINESS because we are talking about our lives, our bodies, our destinies.

ER FOUR - HOW I FOUND OUT ABOUT ...NCIENT SOLFEGGIO SCALE

In Chapter Two, I mentioned receiving an article from a friend about *Healing Codes for the Biological Apocalypse* (1999) by Dr. Leonard G. Horowitz and Dr. Joseph Puleo.[1] The next step in my process was to read this fascinating book and learn about the ancient solfeggio frequencies.

Joseph Puleo is a naturopathic physician currently living in Northern Idaho. Through a series of metaphysical circumstances beginning in 1974, Dr. Puleo was guided into unraveling certain vibrational frequencies and other mysteries encoded in the Bible. He was introduced in a vision to the Pythagorean method of numeral reduction. Using this method, he discovered six sound frequencies hidden in the book of Numbers, Chapter 7, verses 12-89. These frequencies are 396 Hz, 417 Hz, 528 Hz, 639 Hz, 741 Hz, and 852 Hz. The fact that these are significant frequencies was further confirmed when it was discovered that the frequency of 528 Hz was being used in the restoration of DNA. 528 Hz also has a powerful effect upon the water molecules that support the DNA helix. It effects the emergence of beautiful six-sided tetrahedronal lattices discussed earlier in the context of optimal support for DNA functioning.

How Dr. Puleo Deciphered the Six Frequencies

A quick synopsis of how the frequencies were deciphered follows. In the Bible, in the book of Numbers, Chapter 7, verse 12, we find a reference to the *first day*. Moving down six verses, to verse 18, we find a reference to the *second day*. Continuing six more verses, to verse 24, we find a reference to the *third day*, and so forth until the final reference in verse 78 which speaks of the *twelfth day*. What

---

[1] Visit his web page http://www.tetrahedron.org to read about Dr. Horowitz and to order his book.

these verses have in common is that they all refer to a similar idea, or pattern.

To arrive at the first frequency, the actual verse numerals are added using the Pythagorean method of numerical reduction which reduces each numeral to a single digit. Thus, verse 12 is 1+2=3. Verse 18 is 1+8=9 and verse 24 is 2+4=6, verse 30 is 3+0 = 3, verse 36 is 3+6=9 verse 42 is 4+2=6 and continuing in this pattern until verse 78. The pattern here is 3-9-6. 396 is the first frequency, the one named Ut that is associated with the root chakra as taught in the SomaEnergetics techniques.

The next frequency is found by looking at verse 13, which speaks of an offering. Six verses down, in verse 19, the same offering idea is repeated. Six more verses, in verse 25, the offering is again repeated. Thus, by using the Pythagorean method of reduction, we find a pattern has developed. Verse 13 is 1+3=4, Verse 19 is 1+9=10 or l, Verse 25 is 2+5= 7. This pattern is 417, 417, and 417. This is the second frequency. The remaining frequencies are arrived at in the same manner. When all is complete, the six frequencies that emerge are 396, 417, 528, 639, 741, and 852. Refer to *Numbers* Chapter 7 in Appendix A to see for yourself.

In a press release about *Healing Codes for the Biological Apocalypse* by Harvard graduate and public health authority Leonard Horowitz, M.D., he states:

> According to the text, Dr. Puleo was intuitively and spiritually guided to find a pattern of six repeating codes in the Book of Numbers, Chapter 7, verses 12 through 83. When deciphered using the ancient Pythagorean method of reducing the verse numbers to their single digit integers, the codes revealed a series of six electromagnetic sound frequencies that correspond to the six missing tones of the ancient Solfeggio scale. These original sound frequencies were apparently used in the great hymn to St. John the Baptist, along with other Gregorian chants that church authorities say were

lost centuries ago. The chants and their special tones were believed to impart tremendous spiritual blessings when sung in harmony during religious masses. Physicists and musicians alike recognize some of the six tones in this unique interrelated series of electromagnetic sound frequencies that include harmonic sequences similar to those found in The Wedding March.

Professor Willi Apel

As Puleo continued to research the tones, he came across a book titled *Gregorian Chant* (1958) by Professor Willi Apel of Indiana University, who reported that "152 chants are apparently missing. The Catholic Church presumably 'lost' these original chants. These chants were based on the ancient original scale of six musical notes called the Solfeggio (Horowitz 59)."

According to Professor Apel,

> The origin of what is now called Solfeggio ...arose from a medieval hymn to John the Baptist which has this peculiarity that the first six lines of the music commenced respectively on the first six successive notes of the scale. Thus the first syllable of each line was sung to a note one degree higher than the first syllable of the line that preceded it. Because the music held mathematic resonance, the original frequencies were capable of spiritually inspiring mankind to be more 'godkind' (Apel 61)."

I know we do not want to believe that churches and institutions withhold information from us. However, recent discovery of 13 intricately carved angel musicians on the arches of the Roslyn Chapel makes me wonder why anyone would want to hide music? Could it be threatening or dangerous to someone or something? Was it a very special piece that contained magical, harmonic, and resonant properties that resonated in sympathy with spiritual beliefs?

So I went looking for the frequencies and I could not find them within any western instruments. Then I remembered the tuning fork the piano tuner used to get the exact pitch to tune the piano and wondered if I could get the exact frequencies in a set of tuning forks.

What was I to Do with These Forks?

I received my first set of tuning forks through Biosonics. They were constructed based on the frequencies that Dr. Puleo discovered. When I got the forks I wondered what in the world I should do with them. I had read that lute player John Shore in 1711 made the very first tuning fork. He was the lute and trumpeter musician for King William the Third. He used the fork to tune his lute and his trumpet. Of course, that developed into using a fork to tune pianos and other instruments. I could not see how that information could help me now. I was completely unclear about how I would weave these tools into an intelligible protocol for someone to experience a novel source of seed energy for cleansing and revitalizing purposes. What was I to do with these forks?

So I began talking about the science of sound and the frequencies of the tuning forks. I noticed that people were immediately intrigued by the frequencies, what the frequencies meant, and what they could do. I could feel their inner self sit up and take notice. They wanted to know more about the tuning forks. I began to give talks about the tuning forks. One talk was to a big group of senior citizens in California during which I talked excessively long, which usually would cause most seniors to fall asleep or walk out. However, every single person in that room was awake and hanging on every word. They could not get enough of it. They wanted to stay afterwards and continue to talk about the tuning forks.

Playing with the Tuning Forks

Then the inevitable began to happen. People began to ask me to use the tuning forks on them. The ones asking me to do a "tuning" were longtime friends. I felt comfortable and safe to begin to work on them with the forks. I decided just to *play* with the forks. When my inner child heard that word *"play,"* it came alive. The first time I played with the tuning forks on another person was an exhilarating experience. I knew my life was about to change. I was standing at a fork in the road.

The first time I used the tuning forks was between lectures at a retreat center in Ohio. As I prepared to use the tuning forks, I asked my Higher Self, the Divine within me, "What shall I do?" My Higher Guidance said to me, "Do what you know." I thought to myself, "Well, what do I know?" About all I believed at that time, to be scientifically credible, was that, the Mi 528 Hz was being used for DNA repair. I said to the woman, "I am going to check your DNA."

The voice of my Higher Guidance continued, "Use what you have been learning recently." I thought to myself, "What have I learned recently?" I had been learning how the right brain controls the left side of the body, and the left brain controls the right side of the body. The left brain crosses over to be masculine energy on the right, and the right side crosses over to be feminine energy on the left. That means that the left would be the mother's side of the person's life and the right would be the father's side of the family.

I said to the woman, "I am going to check for your dominant DNA." At this point, I felt I could not go back. The fork had enchanted me, calling me along a new and so very resplendent path. This woman was sitting in a chair in front of a group of people watching me and they all trusted me to know what to do. As humans, we are fearful when we are in unknown territory, uncharted waters. We feel so responsible, so helpless. So I had to trust that my Higher Wisdom from within would continue to lead me. The voice came again and said, "Sound the tuning fork on the right side and on the left side and listen with your heart (secret ear)."

When we are doing something for the first time, we have no one to ask, "Is this right?" so we go forward in our fearful and trembling flesh. I did not even know how to properly sound a tuning fork. I just took my shoe off and tapped the tuning fork on the sole of my shoe. The Bible says to take your shoes off when you are standing on Holy Ground. I certainly was, at that moment, in the very much present *now*, standing on Holy (Wholly) Ground.

In fear coupled with great anticipation, I listened for the next instruction. Would it ever come? Was I brought out into the wilderness only to be made a fool? I sounded the tuning fork and held the fork about an inch above the right side of the woman's body. Moreover, it sounded a sound, a very pleasant sound. It seemed pleasant to me, but of course, I had nothing with which to compare it. Then I sounded the tuning fork again, and held it above the opposite side. The sound was totally different. It was louder and more dissonant. The woman sitting on the chair shifted her body. We had connected into some information that seemed to be very strong. Then I heard myself saying: "You have inherited dominant DNA from your father's side, and certain aspects of that dominant DNA are dominant in your personality, not allowing the true person that you are to express."

Now that I had found the dissonance, I wondered "What do I do now? How do I balance it?" Instinctively, I felt the tuning fork moving toward the heart from the dominant side. I had learned that the human system is balanced in the heart. I kept striking the fork until I knew that enough energy from the dominant side had been moved to the heart, and the heart had balanced the right and left sides. I took the tuning fork and struck it again and held it above the right side. It sounded fine. I struck it and held it above the left side, which had been so loud and dissonant and, to my amazement, it sounded exactly like the sound on the right side. I said, "Your DNA is now in balance. You will be able to begin to express your true self now." Later the woman reported that her reactions to experiences were totally being altered. She was beginning to experience lightness within as she let go of old unbalanced, dominate ancestral patterns.

From that first experience with the Mi tuning fork, I began to do regular tunings with the forks, following my Wisdom within. I learned that the forks themselves search and seek out any imbalance and any altered ratios and missing frequencies. The forks restore and repair, heal and balance our systems, bringing us back to the wholeness we were created to be.

As I continued playing with the forks, I began to recognize a definite pattern in the human body's responses to the vibrations created by the different tones of the tuning forks. People began telling me what they felt happening to them and in them. I do not know when it happened, but, soon, a shift happened. I was not using the tuning forks. The tuning forks were using me. It was as though the tuning forks were alive in my hands. They resonated with the energies of the human etheric body. Believe me; they knew one another, like old friends. I found that the body was literally drinking in the tones in nearly desperate gulps to get the life that was being created in the Gap, the Sacred Pause, in the moment. I began to feel that I could trust these ancient tones in the form of tuning forks as a valid sound therapy.

Slowly, but very deliberately, the techniques I now teach in my workshops began to take shape. I treat the tuning forks as though they are conscious "entities." They are energy. They are vibration. They are frequency. The client is vibration, frequency, and energy. I am vibration, frequency and energy. All of that comes together to produce a synergetic experience that takes place on many levels. Use of the tuning forks focuses upon the physical, the etheric, the mental/emotional, and the astral energy bodies.

The tuning forks can search out and find energies of those still in the physical body and those that have left the physical plane. In energy, there is no death. There is just life. During one tuning, the energy of a man's wife who had recently died came forth. Her energy had his energy boxed up and trapped in grief and suffering. Another time I balanced a woman whose father had molested her as a child. She had never told a soul about it, but the tuning fork found that trapped, negative energy that had been controlling her, creating a life based on fear and limitation. The tuning fork also found a flat zone in a woman whose daughter had just been killed in a car wreck two months before her tuning. I never know anything about the person before a tuning session. The tuning forks find the unresolved issues and bring harmony and balance in the physical body.

When we get angry and don't know why, could it be our dominant DNA reacting? Negative patterns stored in the energy body can cause reactions in our daily lives. This energy needs to be repatterned from a reactive to a proactive consciousness. By balancing this energy, we will empower ourselves by allowing our true self to come through in everyday situations.

Development of SomaEnergetics Techniques

My path of exploring and refining these workshops has been validated repeatedly. As I have gone into uncharted territory, there are times when I wonder whether I am on target. Questions constantly came to mind as I started working with the tuning forks. I found that the work is very right-brained, intuitive, and imaginative. The right brain believes to see; the left-brain sees to believe. I felt the need for some left-brain confirmation. I wanted to see some evidence. I needed to see something "scientific" that proved that the tuning forks were actually making a difference.

I was scheduled to speak at a church in North Carolina. A friend living in the area did Kirlian photography. Kirlian photography is the use of a special camera that can photograph the human energy body, called the aura. I called her, and she said she would be doing Kirlian photography that day at a local bookstore. I asked if she could bring someone who did not know me that I could do a tuning on and she could then take a picture before and after the tuning. She brought a lovely woman who agreed to participate in the experiment. My friend took a picture before I did the tuning. Then I did a 20-minute tuning. My friend took another picture. I was amazed at the difference in the woman's energy field before and after the tuning. These photos are available on my website. (www.somaenergetics.com)

After working with the tuning forks for a couple of years, I still asked for more validation. I wanted more proof that I was doing what I was supposed to be doing.

Third Vision: The Missing Stones

I had decided to attend the Annual Sand, Sea, and Spirit Retreat in Gulf Shores, Alabama, to show my tuning forks and give demonstrations. My main purpose for attending the retreat however was my personal intention of receiving validation for my work with the tuning forks. Was I following the right path? Was I doing what I was supposed to do with them?

I decided to go to a meditation held by The Light Weavers who were two ladies, one who played a harp and one who played a flute. The thing that attracted me is that they didn't play any organized music, but played guided by Spirit – creating an atmosphere for people to have personal experiences.

The first time I went into the room, I noticed that the people seemed to be having deep experiences. Therefore, I went back the second day. At the beginning of the meditation, I began to see the most beautiful yellow. I remembered that the color yellow represents wisdom and that wisdom was a feminine energy, sometimes called Sophia by the early Greeks. Then the color began to take on a form. It was a beautiful feminine form, not exactly a woman, but essentially feminine in feeling. She had long flowing gold hair and she was beautiful. I felt that she was Mother Wisdom, a feminine display of The Divine. To the Tibetan Buddhists and Hindus she is Tara. To the Chinese Buddhists she is Kwan Yin. In our predominately Western cultures, which are based in Christianity, we do not presently have an essentially feminine display of the Divine other than Mother Mary who is prayed to in the Rosary in The Catholic Church. But I felt that it was the feminine side of God that I was seeing.

She presided over a sea of glass. As I was observing the beauty of this feminine goddess, I became aware of eyes of concern. As I looked into these eyes across this great sea were six stepping-stones, placed exactly step-by-step, across the sea. The stones were the means for great masses of people to cross the sea from darkness into the Light of all Truth. Each stone was a source of personal enlightenment and self-empowerment. Each stone enabled the person who stepped there to proceed to the next stone until each reached the fullness of all Truth and Wisdom.

As in most visions, the essence of the vision was allegorical and what was envisioned was greater in scope than the size of the vision. In the vision, I instinctively knew that each one of these six stones represented a storehouse of wisdom and knowledge in the Sea of Life. I saw that a person could stay on one of the stones for a long time, even lifetimes, in order to get all of the information that was necessary to proceed to the next stone. In the vision, the people were easily stepping from stone to stone. I also knew these steps were not in time and space, and that the steps reaching from stone to stone in time and space could involve lifetimes.

I also instinctively knew that some people were assigned to certain stones. Their purpose was to teach the wisdom and knowledge of that stone. They had already walked across all the stones and now had come back to be teachers along the path. Each teacher both chose and was assigned to a specific stone.

Then the face of the beautiful feminine Entity began to be troubled. Her beautiful eyes of golden light and love began to cry tears of sorrow. Her eyes followed the actions of certain beings that appeared along the path. Some began to push others off the path into the waters. These beings were clothed in clerical garb. They had on dark hooded robes that jingled and jangled with all kinds of religious paraphernalia, like beads, and crosses and incense burners. They carried small bibles, but the bibles were burning. The words were being burned up, destroyed. Then these beings started removing the stones. The remaining stones were very far apart because some of them were missing. They were so far apart that the people who were trying to cross from stone to stone had to swim in the waters and work very hard to try to get to the next stone. They grew so weary and tired. Some gave up and turned around and went back to the last stone, giving up trying to get to the next stone that was now so far away. They were stuck. They just couldn't go any farther.

Then I saw a stone that had been taken away. It was the stone with the Science of Sound and the truth about the original six creative vibrations. I realized we couldn't go any farther until we know about these frequencies. They are a bridge, a missing stone that takes us to the Realms of Love, Light, and Truth. These missing frequencies will make it much easier to cross over to the next Realm of Life. Life has been so hard for those of us who have been seeking the answers. The journey seemed impossible. With the rediscovery of these frequencies, we have one of the missing stones. Now we can walk across easily to the next part of our path.

I had been calling these missing stones "blind spots in consciousness." Our Universe is missing some of its sounds in the microwave background according to Scientific American (August 2005, 48). As humans, we have blind spots in our consciousness. It may all go back to the missing stones I saw in my vision. Solfeggio is not music, as we know music. These frequencies are vibrational links that fill the blind spots, creating a bridge, so we no longer live in our illusions but we can walk in life with no blindness, no missing notes, playing at the game of Life with all of the tools and pieces we need in order to be healthy, prosperous, successful, and happy.

Vibrational Fields

The laws of Quantum Physics now say that our Universe and everything in it is made up of vibrational fields. Our bodies seem to be solid but are actually patterns of energy vibrating in an immense void. There are many forms of energy besides the human body. For example, plants, animals, and rocks each have different vibrational energies.

Humans have not yet been creative in the fullness of ourselves because so far we have only been producing enough energy to survive. At the deepest level, the level of the super-conscious, we seem to know what to do in our lives, but the majority of us do not do what we know we need to do. As I saw the awesomeness of human potential, I wondered about why we do not use more of that potential. Why stay in an abusive relationship? Why stay in a hated job? People live at this survival level, barely alive, but not getting what they really want from life. SomaEnergetics Level 1 teaches the practitioner how to facilitate the client's chakra system to free up energy. Clients then gain back the energy, become re-vitalized, to make the changes that transform their lives. We are here to be an active part of the total human experience, not just robots that repeat outmoded programs of what already is.

A Recipe for the Universe

As I was returning from a speaking engagement in November 2000, I was struggling with the question of going to nine frequencies as others had done. The three additional frequencies made sense on one level, but there was something holding me back. As I walked through the airport, I saw a *Discover Magazine* that had on the cover the question, "Why Is There Life?" I wanted to relax after a weekend of speaking, but I kept seeing the magazine as I walked to my gate. Finally I purchased the November 2000 issue of *Discover Magazine* and read the article about Dr. Martin Rees and his new book *Just Six Numbers*. Rees says, "Six numbers constitute a recipe for the Universe" (4). He adds that if any one of the numbers were different, even to the tiniest degree, there would be no stars, no complex elements, and no life, as we know it (4).

I am not saying that the six solfeggio frequencies are the six numbers referred to by Rees. This was just a personal confirmation for me to stick with the original six frequencies.

Is it possible that the six days of creation mentioned in Genesis represent six fundamental numbers or frequencies that underlie the Universe? I have always wondered about six being the number of man, as man was brought forth on the 6th day. However, have you considered that in the carbon-12 atom, which is the building block for organic life, there are six protons, six neutrons, and six electrons? This is another way of looking at the number 666.

In Pythagorean numerical reduction, 666 = 9 (6+6+6 = 18. 1+8 = 9) which is completion (the same as 144,000 – 1+4+4 = 9). A woman carries a baby for 9 months and then the baby is birthed as a newly completed, perfect and entirely new human being. Can we now entertain the thought of becoming tuned to a new and perfect human creation?

Realizing Our Ultimate Potential as Human Beings

I hope this information excites you as much as it does me. If you are offering any type of healing work, please consider integrating the tuning forks into your techniques. I see the direction toward healing procedures dealing with frequencies, sound, and color expanding as we head further into the 21st Century. This view is corroborated by many outstanding contemporary scientists and healers. Refer, in particular to *Vibrational Medicine* (2001) by Richard Gerber, M.D, and to The *Energetics of Healing* (2001) by Caroline Myss, Ph.D., best-selling author and medical intuitive. Further, many, including Caroline Myss and Stevin McNamara, have developed specific meditation music that helps to guide and direct energy through the chakras.

I believe that we live in a time of new ideas. Using the tuning forks gives us a way to bypass the resistance of the human ego mind and its powerful collective belief systems. I believe we can touch and expand the heart at its deepest level. This will give us the power to be all that we have the potential to be.

One of the special techniques I teach in my workshops clears the heart chakra and connects it with its highest consciousness of love, light, and truth. This results in an expansion of the heart chakra energy field so we can live more from our heart than from our heads. We then begin to create from our hearts, which contain all solutions to the issues of life. I invite you to be a Co-Creative partner with us as we take this awesome and exciting adventure together.

It has been asserted by many that in a moment, in the twinkling of an eye, anything can happen. It can happen the moment we change our minds. Every breath is an opportunity to change our lives forever. Change precedes transformation. The transformation of the cellular tissue automatically happens when the intent of the mind is focused upon a moment of healing... a moment of peace, of happiness, a miracle moment – a choice point when we are called to choose which *fork in the road* to take.

Where Are the Lightworkers?

I am looking for those who want to work with the new energy and assist others in raising their vibration to the next level of human evolution: HOMOLUMINOUS. I am looking for the people who will help return the missing stones to connect us to the next age. I am looking for the *LIGHT WORKERS,* who are here to learn how to use these tuning forks to fill in the blind spots in contemporary human consciousness. This is the Time. Where are the Workers?

I am looking for those who will work with the interface of the etheric and physical bodies. I want to offer to you, the reader, the idea that we can bring esoteric spiritual experience into life at the physical level with the tuning forks. Perhaps as you read this you will feel called.

This is the new medicine.

In 2000 BC: Here, eat this root.
In 1000 AD: That root is heathen. Here, say this prayer.
In 1850 AD: That prayer is superstition. Here, drink this potion.
In 1940 AD: That potion is snake oil. Here, swallow this pill.
In 1965 AD: That pill is ineffective. Here, take this antibiotic.
In 2000 AD: That antibiotic does not work any more.
  Here, eat this root.
In 2010 AD: That root is contaminated, here,
  practice energy medicine.

Author Unknown

CHAPTER FIVE– ENERGY WORK AND SOMAENERGETICS

So let us now apply these insights to the use of sound frequencies for the body to heal itself. What may manifest as disease in the physical body could be caused by an attachment to some emotion, feeling, or intellectual belief that the person has internalized. Everything that has ever happened, is now happening, or is likely to happen in our lives, is stored in one of our several energy vibrational bodies.

According to Barbara Brennan in her book, *Hands of Light* (1988) it may be in any of the energy bodies. The astral body, which in most people extends from ½ to 1 foot beyond the physical body, contains our actions and reactions in relationships with others. It may be in the next layer, the mental body, which extends about 3-8 inches out from the physical body and contains structures that are thought forms of our ideas. The next layer in is the emotional body, which follows the outline of the physical body and extends 1-3 inches from the physical body, and contains our feelings. Is it in our etheric body, which is ¼" to 2 inches beyond the physical body and pulsates at 15-20 cycles per minute? The Etheric Body contains the prototype of our physical body. This energy continuously becomes our third dimensional physical body (Brennan, 50).

Fifth Dimensional Energy

As mentioned above, beyond the Etheric are other subtle energy bodies that connect us to higher energies. This is the level where life force is still in a more pure, primordial vibration, before it begins the involution process to become matter at the physical level. These subtle energy bodies connect us to fifth dimensional energy. It is the pure and original divine energy coming into our third dimensional experience through the subtle energy bodies. This energy is crucial to the emergence of the new light body. The challenge is that the original blueprint is being aborted by our beliefs and unresolved issues from past experiences, therefore creating energy blockages and resulting in an inferior physical body.

To allow the fifth dimensional energy to create the new light body, we need to bypass the belief systems and clear the energy blockages. There is nothing in our brain right now that identifies with the six Solfeggio frequencies. However, when we tune the subtle energy anatomy, as described by Brennan with the tuning forks, the sounds fire neurons that are not being used and they become places – or portals – for the energy from the perfect divine blueprint to come through our bodies and transform us. When we operate in the fifth dimensional energies, we may directly access inherent human potential to eliminate all disease and eventually death itself.

In the Level I Energy Vitality Technique training using the Solfeggio tuning forks, you can learn to use the vibrations in the coccyx area to activate what I call The Pump – the pump of living waters. In the Upanishads, the final part of the Vedas which are the ancient sacred scriptures of India, this is named the kundalini, sleeping energy or inactive energy at the deepest level of our being. In SomaEnergetics we teach people to awaken the kundalini energy and let it intelligently distribute itself throughout the energy centers, the chakras, to bring the energy from survival level to creative level.

Awakening of the kundalini creates a freedom of sacral motion and harmonic alignment of the sacrum, which can allow for optimal flow of cerebrospinal fluid (CSF). According to John Beaulieu in *Music and Sound in the Healing Arts,* 1987, "CSF is considered by the ancient Taoists to be the physical equivalent of Chi or life energy and, more recently, by cranial osteopaths as the "elixir of life." (92). Dr. William Garner Sutherland, founder of Cranial Osteopathy, has observed that the quality of the cerebrospinal fluid is the basis of health. He states, "Cerebral-spinal fluid is the highest known element in the human body" (Beaulieu, 1987, 92). Tuning with the tuning forks encourages the highest secretion and flow of cerebrospinal fluid. The dural tube that holds the spinal fluid runs from the brain to the sacrum. The spinal fluid is manufactured in the ventricles of the brain. It acts as a shock absorber for the brain and the spinal chord, it supplies the body's central nervous system with nutrients and it disposes of waste products. To the extent that the spinal fluid has freedom to move up and down the tube, where it nourishes and cleanses along the nerve plexuses of the sushumna, it assists in keeping the body healthy.

With the use of tuning forks, the energy, prana or Chi, can be stimulated through vibration up the length of the spine, through all of the chakras. At the top of the head we can create a still point of refraction, before moving down the front to balance all the various systems of the energy anatomy. This process affects all the body's systems: the endocrine, immune, respiratory, reproductive, skeletal, muscular, and autonomic and sympathetic nervous systems. In short, vitality of the entire physiology can occur when one tunes with sound.

Dr. Beaulieu further states, "When we listen to intervals produced by the tuning forks, we stimulate our vestibular nerves. Our vestibular system is the basis of our sense of space, proportion and balance. When we induce a still point with tuning forks, it is hypothesized that the walls of the ventricles (choroid plexus) change their physical proportions to reflect the ratio of the applied interval. The new proportion is optimal for secretion of CSF and balance of the intracranial dural membranes. This in turn harmonically organizes the motion of the individual cranial bones with the sacrum and the sound of the central nervous system." (Beaulieu 1987, 93).

The Solfeggio and Six Precious Metals

According to Sol Luckman[1] in his book, *Conscious Healing* (2005), up to 10 percent of the brain and central nervous system is composed of the following six precious metals: gold, iridium, osmium, palladium, platinum and rhodium. Further, "Kinesiological testing reveals these six metals energetically correspond to, and can be activated by, the six notes of the Solfeggio." (136)

Luckman describes a process whereby activation of our internal chassis of precious metals, stimulates the creation of the light body from within. This internal energy or kundalini, according to Vedic teachings, has the potential to unfold one's compete bio-spiritual enlightenment [the lightbody] when fully awakened. Activating the six precious metals using the Solfeggio frequencies "produces bioacoustic and bioelectric signals capable of turning the body's liquid crystals from hexagons into interlocking tetrahedrons or merkabahs" (Luckman, 137). This concept is reflected in Dr. Masaru Emoto's research showing the metamorphosis that takes place when kind words are spoken to water. You can see the beautiful patterns produced by the Solfeggio frequencies in water molecules on our website – www.SomaEnergetlcs.com.

Energy Dynamics of the Vesica Piscis

Few figures in Sacred Geometry carry so much meaning as the simple Vesica Piscis. The Vesica Piscis (see figure1) is a shape which is the intersection of two circles with the same radius, intersecting in such a way that the center of each circle lies on the circumference of the other. The name literally means the bladder of the fish in Latin. Keith Critchlow has explored this form with great depth and sensitivity in his

---

[1] More information about Sol Luckman and his Regentics Method can be found at www.phoenixregenetics.org.

book Time Stands Still, (1982); however, we will only consider a few of its symbolic interpretations.

One of the symbolic ways to view the Vesica Piscis is as a representation of the intermediate realm which partakes of both the unchanging and the changing principles, the eternal and the ephemeral. Human Consciousness thus functions as the mediator, balancing the two complementary poles of consciousness.

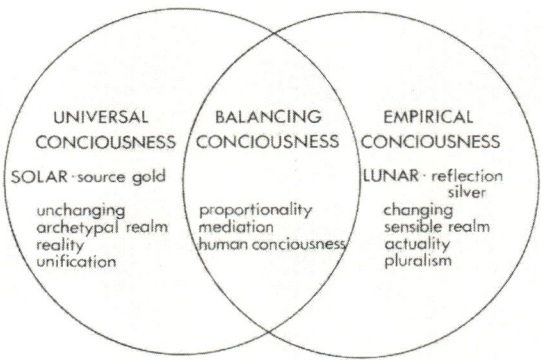

According to Robert Lawler in *Sacred Geometry*, (1982), "The overlapping circles – an excellent representation of a cell, or any unity in the midst of becoming dual – form a fish-shaped central area, which is one source of the symbolic reference to Christ as a fish. Christ, as a universal function is symbolically this region, which joins heaven and earth, above and below, creator and creation. The fish is also the symbolic designation of the Piscean Age, and consequently, the Vesica is the dominant geometric figure for this period of cosmic and human evolution (33)." In the SomaEnergetics Technique, the Vesica Piscis is basically the stillpoint or a portal into all potentiality, all possibilities.

Greg Braden, in *Awakening to Zero Point*, (1997) states that in the Ancient Egyptian mystery schools, the glyph of the eye of Horus (which is actually the Vesica Piscis) represents individual, group, and mass consciousness. Specifically, the right eye of Horus symbolizes the undifferentiated state of awareness. (44) Additionally, it is the Egyptian glyph for the mouth, (as well as for the creator), and is very similar to the Mayan glyph for zero, (which is associated with our galaxy of the Milky Way). Thus, as the forgoing figure highlights, the coming together of Universal (Solar) Consciousness and Empirical (Lunar) Consciousness creates a Balancing Consciousness. (Braden, 147)

A simple Tuning Fork exercise for creating a Vesica Piscis and balancing one's Solar and Lunar frequencies involves utilizing the Sun and Moon Tuners, either in conjunction with the SomaEnergetics Introduction Technique or in a separate tuning.

Thus, as previously stated, in the SomaEnergetics Technique, a Vesica Piscis is formed when there is a sacred pause — when the energies are moved up through the transmitting chakras on the back of the body, to the crown area on the head and are then reversed as the Technique moves the energy down the receiving chakras on the front of the body. The Vesica Piscis is created when the technique changes direction at the crown of the head.

The tuning forks awaken the energy that runs through the many systems of the body. If energy is blocked and not circulating, wherever it is blocked, we experience pain and dis-ease.

The Causes of Aches & Pains

According to The Rev. Marcy Cheek, metaphysician, "An ache is a reaction at the cellular level when the life force energy of the physical body is blocked." She says that the life force energy circulating inside our body all the time is constantly trying to free the "chi" energy and the "pushing" causes the ache. An "ache" is a dull, persistent pain, not a sharp pain. Aches come from yearnings, the yearnings of the soul to return to a balanced state. A yearning is an urgent desire, a desire that has not yet been fulfilled. None of us should ever have aches, because Source has promised to give us all of the desires of our heart. The gruesome fact is we ARE getting all of our desires every day. Since most of us have a high percentage of negative thoughts (psychologists say that 88% of our thoughts are very negative, about ourselves and about others), and these negative thoughts are attached to our desires. Therefore, we get negative circumstances manifesting in our lives and our body aches. The human can invent dozens and dozens of reasons why we can't have what we want – instead of inventing the dozens and dozens of ways that we CAN have what we want. We are using the process, but we need to change the energy that goes into the process. We need to stop being a victim caught in the rushing waters of life at the survival level, being pushed and shoved around by everything and everyone else. We need to get into the Divine DNA-powered boat of our Divine Blueprint and begin to cruise the waters of life. If you've never been on this cruise, now is the time. Learning how to use the tuning forks in all of their proper ratios and probabilities, with imagination, intuition and intention, can get you cruising.

Cheek defines the role of pain in human consciousness:
"Pain is the body recognizing the presence of an unnatural state of imbalance." If we exercise too much and put the body out of balance, we have pain. The body can misinterpret too much exercise as overtaxing our body, which activates the natural process of survival, and the body calls a halt by creating pain.

Level II SomaEnergetics Training is based on the principle that the body is a feedback mechanism. Our body is talking to us all the time. Let us say that there is the experience of knee pain, and it is in the left knee. Left side is the Ying/feminine, receptive side. Right side is the Yang/masculine assertive side. What is the body telling us? Knees represent our willingness to "bend" in life. The knee is below the waist, so it represents a direction we are taking in our lives. This indicates that there is a blockage attached to a thought form connected with a female energy that we do not want to deal with. Beyond this, the tuning fork can search out blockages in the subtle bodies that are still in the thought form stage and change the thought, so it does not then have to manifest at the physical level at all. We can change or eliminate all negative manifestations in our lives. All is possible according to our faith, our intention, and our beliefs.

Speaking of the role of pain in human awareness, Steven Ash in *Sacred Drumming* (2001) says, "Pain makes you move from your comfort zone and seek a solution. It is your choice where you go for this remedy. You may see your pain as not being your responsibility and wish to be a patient (victim) and present your problem to the doctor.... In this way, you have often given away your own power and autonomy. Let us not give away our power. Let us see the pain as a way in which we can move from one chapter in life into another. Pain says, 'Look at me.' It makes you look at things buried down deep in your memories – emotions or beliefs"(28). Pain is the physical body's way of telling us it is out of balance. In some cases, we can use the tuning forks to discover and remove the cause, restoring balance.

If our hearts hurt, there is something that is not supposed to be there. At the beginning of heart trouble, this something could be a thought of hate, revenge, retaliation, regret, jealousy, envy, or anger. Alternatively, it could be an experience of lost love in some way; an experience when someone said or did something that hurt our feelings, betrayed our trust, and violated our integrity. On the other hand, maybe we smoked too much and the blood vessels began to fill up with dangerous and destructive substances. Perhaps we don't eat properly and the vascular system begins to store up too much fat or cholesterol that clogs the flow of blood through the veins and arteries. We can also be influenced by our family's predisposition to heart disease, and since other members of our family have died of heart trouble, we believe that we have the chance of getting heart trouble, too. We introduce these thoughts and these belief systems into our bodies, thus our bodies begin to create heart trouble.

In the SomaEnergetics workshops, we explore the concept that sounds reach deep within to the primordial, plasmatic, bioenergy body where issues of life begin and develop. The plasma body, also known as the energy body, records interactions on a higher cosmic energetic level than the cellular structures. It has no nervous system or rational mind. It is within the cell. It surrounds the cell. It is the cellular memory at a deeper level. Within this plasma substance are responses to previous environments and stimuli that became trapped and , remain active in our everyday lives, sometimes hurting us and sometimes causing us to hurt others. We continue to explore how to use the tuning forks as a modality to expand the energetic periphery and potential of the client to allow for more personal sacred space. I urge you to come to a workshop or get the home study course to learn more of what the tuning forks can do.

The Secret within the Solfeggio Syllables

Ut queant laxis or Hymnus in Ioannem is a plainchant hymn to John the Baptist written by Paulus Diaconus, the eighth century Lombard historian.

Ut queant laxis resonare fibris
Mira gestorum famuli tuorum
Solve polluti labii reatum
Sancte Johannes

In the eleventh century, the music theorist Guido of Arezzo developed a six-note ascending scale that went as follows: ut, re, mi, fa, sol, and la. These Solfeggio Frequencies developed from the first syllables of each line below.

Ut queant laxis
Resonare fibris
Mira gestorum

Famuli tuorum
Solve polluti
Labii reatum
Sancte Johannes

Literal translation of the Latin: "In order that the slaves might resonate (resound) the miracles (wonders) of your creations with loosened (expanded) vocal chords and wash the guilt from (our) polluted lip." This is attributed to Saint John the Baptist.

The expanded and enlarged translations below have been painstakingly written by Gary and Verna Clay, using Latin dictionaries and Webster's Dictionary. Their material from the *Solfa Sound Training Manual*, has been re-printed here with permission.

Expanded translation: "We, as prisoners, are crying out for release from our spoken expression of limited consciousness so that we might resonate with your expanded creative vibrations."

Enlarged translation: "The Divine Mind needs an unconfined and freely moving relationship with us that will resonate our speech, or the very fiber of our being, to produce a miracle of communication, which will solve, dissolve, and release the restrictions of our speech."

Here, "resonate" means to receive larger vibrations that in effect will increase our lower vibrations. Likewise, "resound" means to sound again. We are restoring or remembering our former state of being.

Hidden Meanings in the Frequencies

Looking at the definitions of each of the original syllables, using little known entries from Webster's Dictionary, the original Greek Apocrypha, and Puleo's information, I have determined that these six original frequencies can be used to assist people in opening up their channels of energy (i.e., the sushumna, ida and pingala) to allow the life force energy, Prana or Chi, to flow freely through the chakra system. I believe that this is what the six electromagnetic frequencies were originally supposed to accomplish. Note the particular resonance of each frequency in the following table.

SYLLABLE	FREQUENCY (Hz)	PURPOSE
UT	396	turning grief into joy, liberating guilt & fear
RE	417	undoing situations & facilitating change
MI	528	transformation & miracles, repairing DNA
FA	639	relationship, connecting with spiritual family
SOL	741	solving problems, expression/solutions
LA	852	awakening intuition, returning to spiritual order

The Frequencies and the Chakras

My friend and musician extraordinaire, Lois Winter, developed the following information for me in 2002, based upon my research and distillation of the many sources of information that I discovered on the topic of the Solfa frequencies. SomaEnergetics developed as such a resoundingly strong set of energy protocols because of her loving contribution to my work. This information associates each frequency of the Solfa to frequency, color, element, and intention. See below.

UT - 396 Hz – Root Chakra. 3+6+9 = 18, 1+8 = 9
        Color: Red
        Element: Earth
        Intent: To free and liberate from guilt and fear

RE - 417 Hz – Sacrum Chakra. 4+1+7 = 12, 1+2 = 3
    Color: Orange.
    Element: Water
    Intent: Undoing situations and facilitating change

MI - 528 Hz – Lumbar Chakra. 5+2+8 = 15, 1+5 = 6
    Color: Yellow
    Element: Fire
    Intent: Transformation and miracles/DNA repair

FA - 639 Hz – Thymus Chakra. 6+3+9 = 18, 1+8 = 9
    Color: Green
    Element: Air
    Intent: Re-connecting & balancing

SOL - 741 Hz – Throat Chakra. 7+4+1 = 12, 1+2 = 3
    Color: Blue
    Element: Ether (sound)
    Intent: Expression and Solutions

LA - 852 Hz – Cranial Chakra. 8+5+2 = 15, 1+5 = 6
    Color: Violet
    Element: Consciousness
Intent: Awakening Intuition and Returning to Spiritual Order

The Seventh center is actually the sum of all six chakras functioning in a holistic totality. It is described as a lotus of an infinite number of petals, Thus, the color is white, as it contains all the colors of the rainbow and all of the tuning forks are used at the same time to integrate all centers.

David Hulse, D.D.

SomaEnergetics Frequencies

Our workshops teach how to release the client's energy, to raise the energy beyond that which most people use to just survive. There is an opportunity to consider your own overall consciousness and perfection. We look at the belief systems that generate the thoughts you think. We look at the words you speak, and consider what influences are behind the choices you make, the feelings you feel. and the sense of love and support you experience from others. You may remember actual events in your life, including traumatic experiences, which are stored in cells throughout the body and affect your present well-being. Blockages that have occurred in the physical body caused by these various distortions are rebalanced, returning the body and its systems to a state of homeostasis which is needed for perfect health.

The frequency of the first tuning fork liberates the energy. Therefore, the tuning fork first searches out hidden blockages, subconscious negative beliefs, and ideas that have led to our present situations. These ideas and beliefs actually have mass and can be weighed in a scientific laboratory. Steven Ash states, "Vibrations crack open the shells of limiting thoughts and emotions, establishing order and harmony. The internal organs and tissues love order and harmony and love to be brought into synchronicity and balance" (2001, 29).

The frequency of the second tuning fork produces energy to bring about change. I hear people say, "I need to make a change." "I know I need to get another job." "I know I need to move to a different place." But people don't seem to have the energy to make the changes. It is possible, with the tuning forks, to learn how to use our energy to change what we need to change in our lives. I met a girl in Illinois a few years ago who worked as a massage therapist. She knew she needed to make some changes in her life. Six months after her personal tuning session she called, "I don't know if you remember me, but this is Mary. You did a tuning on me. You will not believe where I am right now. I am in Arizona. After the tuning, I felt enough energy available to me to pack up everything that I own, put it in a truck, and drive to Sedona, Arizona. This had been a dream all of my life." Today she is the head of all massage therapists at a major resort. The tuning forks can put us in touch with an inexhaustible source of energy that allows us to be able to make our dreams come true.

The frequency of the third tuning fork brings transformation and miracles into our lives. We receive clarification, inspiration and revelation concerning our needs, desires, hopes, dreams, and purpose. This frequency activates our imagination, intention, and intuition to operate for our highest and best good.

The frequency of the fourth tuning fork holds electromagnetic frequencies for relationships. Our relationships can be brought into harmony. We are in relationships with our mates, spiritual family, co-workers, service providers, and neighbors. We can live in harmony with these people. We can find co-creative partnerships. Some people find their partners at our workshops. Everything is energy; everything is relationship.

The frequency of the fifth tuning fork leads us into the power of true self-expression, which can only happen after the ancestral DNA is balanced by the third tuning fork. We then begin to be who we really are and to do what we were created to do. In my workshops, many women come who are so dependent upon a male or other authority figure that they can hardly make a sound out of their own being. I take the fifth tuning fork and say, "You represent every woman who has ever been told to be still and not speak, to be submissive to a man or a husband." Often a sound from deep within is released. Women should never let men regulate or control what pertains to a woman. Women need to handle matters that pertain to women. Women need to know to speak up and assume control of their beings. For men, the fifth tuning fork allows the feminine to be expressed and balanced with their maleness.

The frequency of the sixth tuning fork is linked to our ability to see through the illusions of our lives such as hidden agendas of people, places, and things.

The workshops teach how to use all six tuning forks together to produce the frequency that opens the seventh Chakra for divine inspiration, revelation, wisdom, and knowledge. I know of no other healing modality available today that actually produces the seventh sound, as does the use of the six tuning forks. This is the Field. Phonons (sounds) become photons (light) to completely permeate and illuminate the body with light-as-sound, through the principle of refraction. You will learn how to place the forks over the crown chakra to refract sound energy into light energy.

The Life is in the blood. Blood is trapped light. According to the *Keys of Enoch* by J.J. Hurtak., "Frequency attunement will change the physical flesh into...a new garment of light. The blood crystallization levels of ionized consciousness become light through frequency attunement (1977 290-291)."

Level II Workshops

Level II Workshops teach how the tuning forks can be used to map and define the obstacles, or blockages occurring in the etheric body. The tuning fork finds the "cause." Energy Tuning forks do not deal with "effect." They are not a quick fix, such as taking an aspirin to make pain go away. Pain we experience is connected to something at a deeper level of our beings. Through the use of Body Mapping, the tuning fork searches out the cause and begins to allow us to illuminate it so that we may begin to deal with it. It begins to break up the cause. Sound alters matter, changes circumstances and conditions, is the source of physical life, and can rearrange and restore life. Sound travels along the chakra and meridian systems that serve as the body's distribution system of life force energy.

In Level II Advanced Practitioner Workshops you will also learn how to use the tuning forks together in different combinations to produce intervals and ratios to release those old life patterns that no longer serve our present needs, and to balance the energy centers. Level II teaches three specific techniques to open the third eye, balance ancestral DNA, and open the heart chakra.

Level II also explores relationships between the six Solfeggio forks. Three pairs of the tuning forks have an interval of 111 hertz. According to Randy Masters, musical mathematician, in a letter written to me about the solfeggio frequencies, 111 hertz is a universal cell stimulation frequency. In addition, another auspicious interval contained in the six tones is the ratio 741:528. This interval is called a tri-tone and in the early days of music was called the "Devil's Chord." The Catholic Church forbade this interval because it is equivalent to a musical sexual expression that the Church wanted to suppress. You will learn how to create these intervals with the tuning forks in order to produce various known effects that operate in the Universe.

For instance, the Ut (396 Hz) may be tapped with the Fa (639 Hz). The ratio between these is the Golden Mean 1.61364 or divine proportion. Using the Ut and the Fa forks together in this way first frees the energy of the Ut, allowing the Fa fork to bring us into right relationships. Everything is energy. Everything is relationship.

Level III Workshops – Teacher Certification

The Level III Workshop will certify you to teach your own Level I classes. You will be able to purchase supplies from us at a discount and form or complement your existing business by hosting your own workshops.

Purchasing Tuning Forks

SomaEnergetics seminars and workshops present the techniques that have been shown to produce results. We continue to learn about the tuning forks and update you with new information and scientific research that is coming upon the planet today.

In the workshops and seminars, I teach techniques that I have developed over years of working with the tuning forks in all types of situations. Although there are other sources for purchasing tuning forks, the SomaEnergetics tuning forks are manufactured of the highest quality materials and are calibrated exactly according to frequencies of original sounds of Creation as revealed by the personal revelations of Dr. Puleo. My staff and I have been using them for several years now. If you are comparison shopping, carefully check out the source of the tuning forks you buy. Just a simple change in the ratios of the vibrations will not produce the same effect as my precision-made tuning forks. Further, various materials used in the fork construction can affect the quality of the tones.

Things are moving very fast. Are you ready to jump into this exciting Field, this Energy Field, with me NOW, grow, and learn as we go?

You can contact me today by visiting my web site **www.SomaEnergetics.com** or calling 937-912-9229 to arrange, host or attend a training workshop near you. You may also be interested in our six-hour, 4 DVD home study course for the Level I Workshop that is creating great results around the world.

CHAPTER SIX - INTENTION, IMAGINATION & INTUITION

There are three powerful influences for manifestation: Intention, Imagination, and Intuition. Lets explore these three and then I will make a call to you to take responsibility for your health and healing in a way that raises the consciousness of the planet just by your doing so.

Imagination

First, let us look at Imagination. Why do you think we have the ability to imagine? In *The Holographic Universe* by Michael Talbot, physicist David Bohm is quoted, "Imagination and reality are ultimately indistinguishable" (1992, 84). When our brain conceives ideas and thinks about non-material things, imaging and imagining sweet delights or monster possibilities, the brain does not know if those possibilities are real or unreal. It assumes that they *are* real and the body obeys the thoughts. The body can fly through the air in an imagined situation. The body can jump tall buildings in a single bound. We can sit at our desks at the office and swim in the warm waters of Bali at the same time. The events are just as real to the body as if they were being experienced in so-*called real-time*.

Albert Einstein visualized himself riding on a beam of light and imagined what he would experience. This playful experiment with the mind's eye revealed the Theory of Relativity to him. Further, much of what was imagined in early science fiction has now become reality in our modern technological world. Imagination has been given to us to allow us to go beyond the boundaries, go into the limitless and expansive worlds of light and order to consider what might be possible. With imagination, all things are possible. If we did not use our imagination, we would never open up those new worlds of possibility.

So, how does imagination work in the realms of health and healing? Imagination does not mean that we are making something up or denying that it exists. What Einstein imagined actually existed and was later verified by analysis. However, to access it, he used his imagination to penetrate the obstacles imposed by his ordinary awareness and common sense. Our momentary awareness is learned behavior, and is often based on error and wrong concepts. Imagination will take us beyond customary concepts to allow us to investigate and invent new concepts that can then be verified and brought into the common awareness of the many. We begin with our imagination.

Many times, if we are sick, we imagine the WORST. If we have a runny nose, we may quickly imagine that it is pneumonia. We tend to take it to the worst-case scenario. Therefore, we can begin by using our imagination to imagine the BEST. We can imagine the highest and best scenario that could possibly happen. This one action can dramatically change our lives.

Intention

Now let us look at Intention. Webster's Dictionary defines intent in the following way: "firmly directed, having one's attention or purpose firmly fixed. Something intended, a determination to act in a specified way, something done purposely." In Colorado for example, it is solely your *intent* to be married that actually makes your marriage legal. And in most states in the US, one's *intent* is the criteria judges use to decide innocence or guilt.

Think of intent as the main topic that is currently on your mind. It is the mind's energizing force to create or change something. Intent is the purpose and the goal behind an idea or desire. Intent has emotion. Emotion is the energy of intent. Emotion is the impulse or force that activates intention. Whatever emotion is connected to the intent is communicated through the choice of action and brings a corresponding result. According to Johnathan Goldman, in *Healing Sounds* (1992) speaking about the relationship between sound and emotion, action and intent, musician Steven Halpern, Ph.D., shared with him: "Sound is a carrier wave of consciousness" (18). This means that depending upon where an individual's intent is placed when he or she creates a certain sound, the sound will carry subliminal information to the person receiving it. For example, if you are angry and you create a sound with a musical instrument or in conversation, it might sound pleasant, but you will be sending anger that is incorporated in that sound.

Researchers have demonstrated that intent has molecular consequences, cells have receptors, and memory and intent vibrate these receptors. Robert V. Gerard says in his DNA Activation Workshops, "It is my conviction that intent is the highest form of creation given to mankind. Our God-given right to utilize free will and choose is preceded by our intent." Intent can determine the types of choices and the types of results we get from our choices. Gary Zukav, best-selling author of *The Seat of the Soul*. (1999), agrees. He says, "Every experience and every change in your experience reflects an intention. An intention is not only a desire. It is the use of your will" (106). Like it or not, every intention that we create also creates the life scenario to follow. Therefore, imagination and intent are extremely important in dealing with health and well-being. Moreover, imagination and intent are extremely important in working with the tuning forks.

Intuition

Finally, Intuition. The third "I" at work in you. Our intuition is our Higher Self, or God Self. So many times in my life, I've heard this *voice*. It sometimes is at the tip of my shoulder. It sometimes is right inside the outer rim of my ear. It is the *still, small voice* of the Intelligent Energy that imbues everything. It knows all. It incorporates all things in its wisdom and understanding. It is never wrong. It is always right on. Have you ever heard yourself say, "If I had only listened to that voice." Intuition is the voice that leads and guides, giving us information that is for our highest and best good. Usually, the message is so positive and so high in love and wisdom that we discount it because it does not fit our everyday habitual struggle for existence. It seems too easy. However, if we could get into the flow of the intuition that is always there, is always right, is always awake, alert, and aware of everything, we could have fantastic lives. . . .lives full of love, power, health, and happiness. So, get in touch with the soft, subtle voice of your intuition.

All who aspire to become co-workers and healers with Soma-Energetics™ working with energy at the cellular level using the tuning forks, need to be in touch with their intuition. Your intuition works synergistically, together with the intuition of the client, to lead you-the-practitioner to tune the client with the frequencies that he or she most needs.

Our ego-mind will question everything that we try to do. It will be full of warnings and memories of other times and other places when emotionally laden, mostly unpleasant, experiences attached themselves to us. The ego-mind can only work according to the information that has already been programmed into it. That may not be enough when we are moving into the limitless and boundless worlds of life and health and peace.

So few of us even know about these realms of intuitive awareness that we have no information already stored about them in our brains. So we will have to rely upon intuition, the source of all Truth and Wisdom. As learners, we are not used to relying on our intuitive, imaginative selves. We often let analytical thinking squeeze out all room for intuition, closing our availability to receive this *voice of imaginative freedom*. Most education in our society focuses on left-brain logical skills, largely at the expense of right brain creative skills. When a premium is placed on analysis, deductive reasoning, and logic, then intuition, insight, and imagination take a back seat and may even be denigrated or punished as methods to distill information from the ether about what is REAL. This is a paradoxical situation, since most of the great scientific discoveries have occurred because of insight and intuition rather than analysis and deductive reasoning. Thomas Edison placed himself in a hypnotic trance-like state to bring forth his most important inventions. Crick and Watson played with Tinker Toys in their discovery of the structure of DNA. Einstein knew this, using an oft-quoted mantra of "intuition first, analysis later."

Many of the skills needed to use the tuning forks reside more within the subjective or unconscious realm. As you become acquainted with your tuning forks and practice with them, you will begin to feel and hear the subtle differences that occur, intuit what is going on, and become able to use them to balance a client's energy field based upon the client's energetic intelligence. Don't focus too much on the analytical, left brain side of learning. If you do, you will hear things like, "Did I do it right?" or "Is this really happening?" There is no right or wrong in intuition. There is only action. Intuition brings focus to intention that then directs the energy in a truly imaginative and creative way. Further, it is important to remember that INTUITION ALWAYS TRUMPS TECHNIQUE.

These three "I"s illustrate the power of intention to manifest form. Truly, as David Bohm says, "Every action starts from an intention in the implicate order. The imagination is already the creation of the form, it already has the intention and the germs of all the movements needed to carry it out, and it affects the body, and so on, so that as creation takes place in that way from the subtle levels of the implicate order, it goes through them until it manifests in the explicate. [. . .] Images in the mind can ultimately manifest as realities in the physical body" (Talbot 1992 84).

Intuition, then, brings to our visualized heart's desires ways to attain them, allowing Co-Creative manifestation to occur and bless our lives. Let us, as powerful spiritual beings, perfect and refine our human experience, using our imagination, intent, and intuition.

/O – THE SCIENCE OF SOUND

CHAPTER SEVEN - MUSICAL SYSTEMS

In *The World is Sound* (1991), Joachim-Ernst Berendt says that the 12-Tone Equal Temperament mistunes all consonant intervals except the octave. 12-Tone Equal Temperament is a limited and *closed system*. Substituting 12 equally spaced tones for a vast universe of subtle intervallic relationships virtually painted music into a corner from which it has not, yet, extricated itself. 12-tone equal temperament can create situations such as 'boxed-in' thinking, stuffed and suppressed emotions, fear-based or lack consciousness, all of which then tend to manifest into physical symptoms called 'dis-ease' or disease.

All of us, including our children, are subjected everyday to the 12-Tone Equal Temperament mentality that produces an overly busy, caffeine high, nervousness. Our society's solution is to put everyone on tranquillizers or Attention Deficit Disorder (ADD) medications. We put the kids on drugs and they listen to Western music. Imagine what would happen if we put earphones on them and fed their delicate auditory systems music played in Just Intonation, by composers such as Mozart. Miracles are happening when kids listen to Mozart's compositions using Just Intonation.[1] People in our society are starved for the primordial sounds of Creation, the exact ratios and frequencies as they were first sounded forth. According to Stuart Isacoff, author of *Temperament: The idea that Solved Music's Greatest Riddle* (2001), 12-Tone Equal Temperament "is a violation of nature. It is like throwing away the key to the universe (17)."

This change in the way all instruments are tuned has affected all human consciousness. According to David B. Doty, in *The Just Intonation Primer* (1993), "Although it is difficult to describe the special qualities of Just Intonation

---

[1] Refer to http://www.tomatis.com

intervals to those who have never heard them, words such as clarity, purity, smoothness, and stability come readily to mind. The supposedly consonant intervals and chords of the 12-Tone Equal Temperament sound rough, restless or muddy in comparison." From pure, clear, and smooth to rough, restless, and muddy.

David B Doty goes further to present the idea of consonance, one particular feature of Just Intonation: "the simple-ratio intervals [. . .] are 'special relationships' that the human auditory system is able to detect and distinguish from one another and from a host of more complex stimuli. They are what the human auditory system recognizes as consonance."

Consonance

Musical compositions based on the 12-Tone Equal Temperament tuning cause this consonance, with the exception of the octave, to deviate significantly from the optimal, integer-ratio forms. The "virtues of Just Intonation and the shortcomings of equal temperament are not limited to the affective properties of their respective intervals and chords. It also deprives composers and theorists of the means for thinking clearly..." (Doty 1994) This might sound strange, but it says something vitally important. What I hear is that 12-Tone Equal Temperament compositions tend to affect our ability to think clearly and deprive us of the means for maintaining close relationships with others and with our environment.

Music and vibration are mysterious and wonderful; there is more than one type of sound. There are consonant notes and dissonant curves. A pure tone sounds only at a fundamental frequency, or pitch. Musical tones are complex in that they not only sound at the fundamental pitch, but also at higher resonant frequencies sometimes-called overtones. I call this The Field. Transposing a piece of music to a new key can completely change its character.

You can tune an instrument like a piano with a result that it has equally mistuned intervals, with no interval grossly out of tune, but none in perfect tune because they must be relative to each other. If you have ever tried to tune an autoharp, you will learn the truth about tuning. As my piano tuner said, "It will NOT be in tune, the chords have to be 'adjusted' so they will fit together, especially the major third."

The Hand of God Tunes the World

Since many of us listen to music every day of our lives, let us look at the bigger picture of what is going on with possibly one of the largest fields of influence upon humanity today. I would like to quote Ruth Franklin who is reviewing Stuart Isacoff's book *Temperament: The idea that Solved Music's Greatest Riddle*

Even if a key to the universe could be discovered, the lock that it fits has long ago disappeared. But for thousands of years, from the ancient Greeks to the original Church fathers of enlightenment, the existence of such a key ... was situated at the intersection of music, science (physics and mathematics), and religion. (Powells 2001)

The proportions that govern musical harmony, causing certain tones that vibrate together to produce a beautiful sound, were believed to agree with the sounds and motions of the celestial bodies. These proportions – simple ratios built on the integers 1, 2, 3 and 4, were proof of the divine organization of the cosmos. As Stuart Isacoff succinctly puts it: "The hand of God tunes the world" (Isacoff 156). Can you believe it? We are resonating with all of the celestial bodies. Haven't you ever wondered why your heart leaps when you see the full moon?

The priestly musicians of Egypt or Mesopotamia are credited with the development of both mathematics and religion in these ancient societies. Pythagoras of Samos is generally credited with introducing whole number-ratio, or integer-ratio, tunings. Pythagorean tuning is characterized by consonant octaves, perfect fourths, and perfect fifths, based on ratios of the integers 1, 2, 3, and 4 with all other intervals, including thirds and sixths, being treated as dissonances.

Jeremy Narby, author of *The Cosmic Serpent* (1999), explains that the author of the Sherlock Homes Investigations, Conan Doyle, wrote that "Sherlock Holmes would lock himself in his office and play dissonant tunes on his violin late into the night – only to emerge the next morning with a key to the mystery" (47). To the western musically trained ear the Solfeggio tones sound dissonant. This dissonance opens the mind to more subtle levels of information.

The Ut Note?

The original musical scale had six tones, beginning with Ut, then Re, Mi, Fa, Sol and La. When I first read this, I thought to myself, "I've never heard of the Ut note. What happened to it." Then one day, someone brought me a classical CD she found at a garage sale and, lo and behold, I found a piece of music written by William Byrd, English composer, 1543-1623 titled "Ut, Re, Mi, Fa, Sol. There it was. The Ut note. Byrd had used it. I wondered if Beethoven and Mozart did, too. In those days, remember, tuning was done differently from today's 12-Tone Temperament based on A-440.

Ruth Franklin writes,

> Pythagoras's theory of the ratios for octaves and fifths was a small subset of his general conception of the Universe, which he perceived as defined by mathematics. The proportions of the musical intervals, like the laws governing geometric shapes and the laws directing the movements of the planets, were all part of the natural order of the

cosmos, all of which had certain simple mathematical formulas. The musical formulas reflected the vibrations of man's nature, which Pythagoreans called 'musica humana' or the continuous soundless music produced by each human being, which would be harmonious or disharmonious with the music of the heavenly spheres as they moved in their orbits. In the vastly thrumming Universe, the vibrations of man's nature and the harmony of the celestial spheres resonated together in sympathetic vibration. (Powells 2001)

Isn't this amazing. Not only do the organs inside of our bodies hum together as they vibrate in resonance, but our bodies also hum along together with all of the celestial spheres. The cosmos is one great big music machine and most of us are out-of-tune with it. Can being tuned with the Solfeggio Frequencies tune our bodies with the cosmos?

The August 2005 issue of *Scientific American* includes an article titled "Is The Universe Out Of Tune?" that discusses the sounds of the Universe which scientists call the cosmic microwave background. It seems that there are some parts missing. They describe the Universe as bodies of sound sitting in the sky as musicians sit together in an orchestra. In this article, the scientists say we are missing the bass and the tuba.

In *The World is Sound* (1991), Joachim-Ernst Berendt also acknowledges that since the time of Pythagoras, such sages and scholars as Plato, Cicero, Philo of Alexandria, and later Johannes Kepler, have known that each planet in our solar system generates a certain tone. Berendt says,

> For millions of years, longer and more steadily than any other comparable vibration, the earth, sun, moon and the planets have been vibrating in cosmic space. Our genes and those of all living beings have experienced these vibrations so often

that the processes and mechanisms of genetic programming have stored them long ago.

Late sixteenth century philosopher Johannes Kepler (1596-1611) said sound is the *verissimae Harmoniae* archetype, *qui intus est in Anima,* or "the archetype of the truest harmony which lies within our soul." Berendt continues, "When we hear these primordial tones, we recognize them as old friends." We incorporate Planetary Tuners[1] within our spectrum of protocols because of the unique attribute that each planet's frequency can invoke creating a sympathetic resonance between the planets and ourselves: Sun for strength, Mars for motivation Jupiter for trust, etc.

A Hertz Makes A Difference

We humans began messing around with the intervals. We changed the ratios. Since Earth is a free will planet and we can do whatever we want to do here, we messed around. This is how that original Mi note at 528 hertz was altered to a Mi note that is now only 512 hertz. We went from beneficial, ENLIVENING Gregorian chants based on an original scale of creative power, in harmony with God and the Cosmos, to a noisy rock and roll concert of self-abnegation and often despair. And the world has been in chaos ever since.

We boxed up the sound in 12-Tone Equal Temperament to invent a way we thought would be more harmonious. What happened is that we closed the vertically spiraling, boundless melody of the Field of All Possibilities that had been sung by the Creator. We lost the key to the Universe's power to create and change, to alter and to repair matter. Music became a method to separate us from our God source. Music became a tool to manipulate and control rather than to soothe, to heal, to bring joy out of sorrow, to dissolve guilt and fear. Music was no longer a tool to raise human nature and the human mind to higher frequencies. It

---

[1] You can explore these Planetary Tuners at http://www.somaenergetics.com.

was no longer a means into the nature and mind of God, a method to bring harmony and a quorum of agreement, or a tool to find the answer to a riddle and to heal and to produce miracles.

Your Secret Ear

Do you know that your *secret ear* can calculate exact ratios between frequencies? It can, and with astonishing accuracy. "Way down upon the Swanee River" is E, D, C, E, D, C, C', A, C' – or mathematically, 5/4, 9/8, 1/1, 5/4, 9/8, 1/1, 2/1, 5/3, 2/1. That secret, or intuitive, ear can detect sounds out of the range of our five senses, and most of the great composers used the secret ear to write their music. According to biographer, Eric Bloom, Beethoven had to use his *secret ear* because in his natural ears, he was deaf. Beethoven was not a church-goer, but avidly studied the Bible and Eastern mysticism. Beethoven acknowledged God as the source of his music. He believed that he had been "called as an agent" to spread the Divine message. Beethoven, like his friend and messianic mentor, Mozart created his masterpieces by transposing the mathematics encoded in the Bible and elsewhere into musical scores. (Horowitz 1999)

According to Alfred Tomatis, M.D., a leading French otolaryngologist who developed the science of Audio-Psycho Phonology (APP), the way we hear has a profound impact on almost all aspects of our being. In his research, he discovered that nearly all the cranial nerves lead to the ear. Dr. Tomatis says that the ear is particularly related to the vagus or 10th cranial nerve. (Tomatis 2001 – 2008) This nerve affects the larynx, the bronchi, the heart and the gastro-intestinal tract, and thus, our breathing, our heart rate and our digestion. No wonder sound has such altering and changing effects.

David Hulse, D.D.

Finding the Key to the Universe

So, what do we do now? How can we get back to those original tones that will allow us to reconnect with the higher dimensions and find healing and health and well-being, harmony and agreement, for ourselves and our earth? What is the missing link? How do we find the key? According to the great father of electromagnetic engineering, Nicola Tesla, "If you only knew the magnificence of the 3, 6 and 9, then you would have a key to the Universe.."

The 3, 6, and 9 are fundamental root vibrations of the Solfeggio frequencies in the tuning forks used in my SomaEnergetics workshops. Come with me now into the science of sound. The Realms of Love and Light can be created with tuning forks tuned to the ancient Solfeggio.

Since most music in our contemporary world – from commercials to modern hymns and symphonies, has been composed utilizing the 12-Tone Equal Temperament Scale, it all has vibrational limits. It creates boxed-in thinking, promotes emotional suppression, and fear-based consciousness centered upon scarcity. This is in contrast to music created from the ancient Solfeggio frequencies, which stimulates expanded creativity and facilitates problem solving and holistic health.

One of the best ways to open the cells of our body so that the messages can be transmitted to the DNA is by sound. Given that our bodies are composed of approximately 78% water, and that sound has the potential to organize and re-pattern matter, we can alter and change anything and everything in the so-called physical world just by our deliberate, intentional, observation of it.

Lee Lorenzen, Ph.D., has invented a patented process that introduces a high level of electromagnetic power (sound) into ordinary water, causing it to cluster in beautiful six-sided crystals. Recall that clustered water can move freely through the cell walls and transport nutrients, remove waste, and help to maintain proper communication between the cells. Even the DNA in each of our cells is folded around a core of this clustered and highly organized water (Horowitz. 1999, 180). Biochemist Steve Chemiski says the 6-sided clear clusters that support the DNA double helix vibrate at a specific resonant frequency – 528 hertz – my Mi tuning fork. The tuning fork can be used to cluster water and nourish our cells, and every cell holds our DNA (Horowitz 1999, 180). These authors are in concert with my message that nothing is set in Stone. Stone can be altered and changed.

Let's look at what others have discovered and written concerning the science of sound.

CHAPTER EIGHT - THE SCIENCE OF SOUND & VIBRATIONAL HEALING

"What if all of animated nature be but organic harps diversely formed, that tremble into thought as o'er them sweeps...one intellectual breeze...at once the soul of each and the God of all?" Samuel Taylor Coleridge (Poem: The Eolian Harp 1795).

Sound can energize us when we are tired. Sound can soothe us when we are upset. Sound can lift our spirits when we are depressed. Sound can comfort us when we are grieving. Sound can heal us when we are sick. Sound can relax us when we are tense. Sound can redirect the innate, divine healing energy within us to wherever it is needed most and in the exact way it is needed. Sound is divine in that it knows only to operate according to the original principles of life and health, according to the Divine Blueprint held in each human's etheric body. Sound works according to divine ideas. Sound activates the Divine in us and works only in perfection – perfectly. Life is vibration. Vibration creates sound.

We can look back at the ancient cultures of Japan, China, Tibet, and India where energy work was considered to be a natural part of health and healing for information that resonates with the knowledge of vibrational healing. This information aligns with what is being said and discovered today about the body's entire electrical "wiring system."

In these ancient systems three primary energy channels control the body-electric, the sushumna, the ida, and the pingala. Each will be discussed in turn in the text that follows.

The Sushumna is the central channel running vertically through the body, along the spinal column, from the Crown to the Root Chakra. On the physical level, this correlates to the brain and spinal cord of the central nervous system. On the etheric level, the chakras are located along the Sushumna line, while distinct from it.

The Ida & Pingala are a pair of moving energy channels located on either side of the Sushumna. They are sometimes referred to as the Shakti and Shiva. They move in an intertwining path along the Sushumna and every place these energy paths cross over, an energy vortex, or chakra, is created.

The pingala is the masculine energy current. The ida is the feminine energy current. The crossover point where the Ida and Pingala change directions is called the Yukta Triveni (meaning combined three streams). It is located at the perineum point, which is found in the area between the anus and genitals. The Pingala originates at the left side of the perineum and teminates at the left nostril; the ida originates at the right side of the perineum, terminating at the right nostril. SomaEnergetics tuning fork sessions stimulate, balance, and integrate the masculine and feminine energy currents.

In order for energy to flow at all, there must first be a "charge." As authors Peggy Dubro and David Lapierre, write in *Elegant Empowerment* (2002), "to charge means to influence, alter, or imprint with a pattern of information (239)." Dubro says, "The ability to rearrange these energy charges creates an opportunity for release, often known as a karmic release, from restrictions of the past. I like to refer to this ... as a 'state of grace'" ... (69). I call this "The Sacred Pause.

Let us continue to explore what has been said and what continues to be said today about the science of sound from many different perspectives.
Following is a compilation of material that has come to me over the years that supports my contention of the importance of Sound Healing at this time. Some of it has come in the form of email or copies with no reference

information. I have cited the original material where possible.

Alice Bailey

According to Alice Bailey, a metaphysician at the turn of the last Century who was way ahead of her time, 'sound, light, vibration and form blend and merge" (1993). She called this

> the blending of the hierarchies – the myriad of energies and frequencies that are constantly intermingling with each other.. Sound permeates all forms of creation. The planet itself has its own note. Each atom has its sound. All humans have their unique chords and all chords contribute to the great symphony, which the celestial Hierarchy and humanity are playing.

Bailey comments specifically upon the meaning of the emergence of this symphony from the perfection of silence.

Through the medium of sound, God spoke and the worlds were made. It has been said that the chief agency by which Nature's wheel is moved in a phenomenal direction is sound, for the original sound sets in vibration the matter of which all forms are made and initiates that activity which characterizes even the very atoms of substance. First the sound, then the pouring forth of Light and then the form.

Alice Bailey ends her dissertation with a prophecy – and remember, this was prophesied before the turn of the last Century:

> The response of the human mechanism to the world of sound will cause developments that will usher in a new age. It will be an age…in which the work of the world will be carried forward through the medium of sound, and eventually using words of power and the efforts of trained sound workers. These trained

workers, understanding the nature of matter and comprehending the purpose of sound will bring about those structural changes and those material transformations which will establish a civilization of a new race.

Healing by the means of sound will be one of the first modalities to be noted in the coming periods. The world is on the verge of entertaining a new era in scientific discovery. An entirely new language related to energy and force is already in the making, and the handling of disease in the immediate future will be little short of the miraculous. The new and coming technologies will throw light on ancient formulas. The physical body will be realized as an electrical unit. The energy body, the etheric vehicle, the explosive nature of energy when it is in contact with force, will be revealed.

Every sound is distinguished by a specific color, a particular tone, a special form, a degree of energy or activity, and the nature of the ensouling life. The man who has spiritual intuition, purity of life and heart, altruistic intentions, self control and courage will be given the power to further the purpose in the work of evolution.

Cathie Guzette

Poet Cathie Guzzetta summarized this science best when she wrote, "The forms of snowflakes and faces of flowers may take on their shape because they are responding to some sound in nature. Likewise, it is possible that crystals, plants and human beings may be, in some way, music that has taken on visible form" (1991, 149).

Guiliana Conforto

In *Man's Cosmic Game* (1998), Guiliana Conforto says, "Every cell of matter is pulsating, reflecting and interacting with every other cell of matter, whether it is in you or in the galaxy. The earth and the sun vibrate in unison based on the main rhythm of 160 minutes. DNA has its own melody. The vibratory nature of all energy can be balanced and put into unison."[1].

Dale Pond

Dale Pond gives us an in-depth look at how the whole Universe, is really music. Apparently, we were truly sung into existence. Haven't you always wondered why you get along with some people and not with others? Is it because some people are in our chord of music and others aren't? It's really simple. You might be a C major chord person. So you will get along great with other C major chord people and probably with G major chord people and F major chord people. But you won't "sound" right or resonate and feel in harmony with B flat minor chord people or even G sharp major chord people.

In *Universal Laws Never Before Revealed:Keely's Secrets* (1995) . Pond combines scientist Walter Russell's statement, "The universe consists solely of waves of motion," with scientist John Keely's Law of Sympathetic Vibration. "All vibration is intimately connected to all other vibration...which demonstrates the interconnectedness of all things and all energies, from simple vibrations to complex chords." Pond says that vibrations are "living things." "They are creative and evolutionary simultaneously. They are active and prolific in their dynamics as are their harmonic offspring."

The "C" Family Gene

Pond continues this fascinating discussion by actually calling these different chords the "C" family gene. Or the "G" family gene. I love it. Wouldn't you rather have a "C" family gene according to the Divine Blueprint for Creation than those

---

1 http://www.giulianaconforto.it/English/home.Eng.htm

genes you got from your parents? We can be tuned to vibrate according to the *original* family gene pool of the *original* Divine Blueprint for Creation. Sometimes all we need is a good tune-up.

Geopathic Stress

Sound is being experimented with today to reduce geopathic stress. Geopathic Stress or harmful earth rays is natural radiation that rises up through the earth and is distorted by weak electro-magnetic fields created by subterranean running water, certain mineral concentrations, fault lines and underground cavities and claimed by some to have a 92% correlation to cancer and other illnesses. In Cape Town, South Africa, pollution of the area called Cape Flats decreased 50% within hours of doing a ceremony that utilized special sonic vibrations through a series of harmonizers in the area. I am indebted to Christan Hummel[1] for this information. Her article, "Sound, The Key to Ending War and Pollution?" appeared in the November 2002 issue of *Sound Magazine*.

She also shared, "In ancient times, Brahmin priests performed a ritual called Agni-hotra, using chanting of certain tones to produce vibrations in the ethers, now called atmosphere, considered beneficial to the planet's well-being. It has been scientifically documented that this process lowers pathogenic viruses and bacteria.".

Do you wonder why we have not applied this information regarding the use of sound to end the problems on Earth today? Do not wonder any longer. The issues at stake in protection of the status quo are money, politics, and control. To use sound to eliminate viruses and bacteria would destroy most of the trans-national corporations and businesses in our society. Nearly our entire global economy

---

[1] Refer to Christan Hummel's website for more information: http://www.earthtransitions.com/content/intro.html.

infra-structure is built upon a foundation of illness, sickness, and death.

Royal Raymond Rife

Scientist Royal Raymond Rife discovered that the unique electronic signature of each specific disease could be modified, rapidly and harmlessly, to eliminate a multitude of known human afflictions. His discovery identified that every single biochemical compound vibrates at its own distinct frequency pattern. Therefore, every living thing has its own unique electromagnetic signature, and this pattern or vibration is unlike any other species or organism. Just as the resonant frequency that shatters a wineglass can only shatter a certain type of glass, so too, Rife's frequencies destroy, or neutralize, only disease organisms with exactly the same pattern of that disease organism. His frequencies destroy viruses with their own frequencies – using frequencies to cancel frequencies in illustration of the adage *like attracts like*.

Raymond Rife understood that viruses and bacteria all have their own etheric fields and the field must be destroyed or the virus will reconstitute itself. So he created a field of resonance and hit the target bacteria or virus with its specific field of sound, destroying the virus or the bacteria. With tuning forks, the field can be produced. Using the Solfeggio frequencies produced by the tuning forks in the etheric part of the body we resonate in the Field. Within the field are all the levels of the body's creation.

We can now go into the depths of the body's systems, beyond the realm of drugs, surgeries, or even acupuncture. Today, we are in the process of re-discovering these truths. We have the power to now apply them to ourselves without outside powers keeping us isolated, sick, diseased, and penniless.

Chladni Sand Figures

Ernst Chladni, musician and physicist, did extensive research into the science of sound. The November 1989, issue of *Sound and Vibration Magazine*, published an outstanding article on Chladni wave plate modes and frequencies. Chladni developed a technique that demonstrates how sound waves affect physical matter. He drew a violin bow across the edge of flat plates covered with sand. The vibration produced geometric patterns and shapes in the sand that are today referred to as "Chladni figures," proving beyond all shadow of doubt, that sound affects physical matter. This action of vibration on matter later became known as "cymatics" after the Greek word for "wave." Today cymatics is defined as the study of how vibrations, in the broadest sense, generate and influence patterns, shapes and moving processes. The Chladni sand figures appear there, showing that for every sound a corresponding shape or pattern can be seen – literally made visible through vibration. In 1815 mathematician Nathaniel Bowditch followed up on Chladni's discoveries. He concluded that conditions for the appearance of these designs depends upon frequencies, or oscillations per second, occurring in whole number ratios to each other – such as 1:1, 1:2, 1:3 and so on.

According to John Beaulieu, in *Music and Sound in the Healing Arts*, (1995), "Form is the more elusive component of sound. Sound-forms can be seen by subjecting mediums such as sand, water or clay to a continuous sound vibration" (1995, 37).

Hans Jenny

The following pictures taken by Hans Jenny are sound-forms. They were obtained by placing various media on a steel plate with a crystal sound oscillator attached to the bottom. The oscillator creates a pulse that vibrates the steel plate.

The forms on the plate are examples of sound organizing and re-patterning matter.

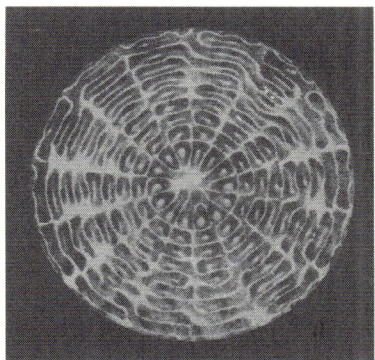
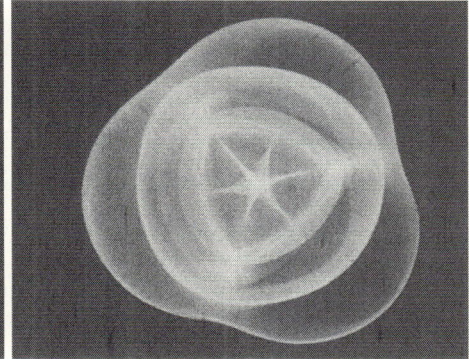

Jenny also noticed that when the vowels of ancient languages like Hebrew and Sanskrit were pronounced, the sand took the shape of the written symbols for those vowels. Modern languages, including English, failed to generate those patterns. Jenny concluded that there are examples of cymatic elements and their effects and actions everywhere, and that these vibrations, oscillations, pulses, wave motions, pendulum motions, rhythmic courses of events, and serial sequences affect everything, including biological evolution. The evidence convincingly demonstrated to him that all natural phenomena are ultimately dependent on, if not entirely determined by, the frequencies of vibration. He argued that different frequencies influence genes, cells and various structures in the body. He claimed that physical healing could be aided or hindered by vibrational tones..

Dr. John Beaulieu

According to Dr. John Beaulieu, naturopathic physician, polarity therapy practitioner, and classically trained musician, as well as a doctor of counseling:

> All sounds are potentially music. When we learn to use our ears to "feel," something very special begins

to happen. You feel pulsations, and from pulsations you can begin to sense rhythm, and from rhythm you can see lights. The pulse, rhythms and lights you tune into are going to affect your thinking, body posture, emotions, and what you allow (or don't allow) into your life.

The more diverse your listening abilities are to different sounds, the more diverse your life becomes. Feeling through hearing can turn into a vibrational experience. As energetic beings, we can begin to pulsate at different frequencies to become more flexible and spontaneous – which translates into wellness. When there is no flexibility or spontaneity, we say there is an energy block (or no dissipation of energy), which will ultimately lead to dis-ease (without harmony).

Dr. Beaulieu reminds us that our mission is to learn to resonate with whatever comes into our lives. Dr. Beaulieu, is the developer of "BioSonic Repatterning." [1] "BioSonic Repatterning" means "life sound." This modality, as a branch of energy medicine, uses music and sound to enable clients to tune into and align their natural rhythms with their individual life sound. The process includes the use of tuning forks plus other modalities such as dance and movement, color and light, flower essences, and dowsing. The principles of this theory can be used to interface with and enhance craniosacral balancing, communication, nutrition, and consciousness exploration. I want to take this opportunity to thank Dr. Beaulieu for his support and mentoring as we have developed SomaEnergetics.

Dr. Andrew Weil

I heard Andrew Weil, M.D., a leader in the field of integrative medicine, and leading authority on brainwaves and

---

[1] More information can be found at www.biosonics.com.

healing, say on the Oprah Winfrey Show, "The body knows how to heal itself." We just need to get all of the old thought systems and untruths we have been taught that limit us out of the way and let the body do what it already knows how to do. Dr. Weil has produced an outstanding CD titled "Sound Body, Sound Mind: Music for Healing" which presents an hour of symphonic sounds guided by the principles of "psychoacoustics," a scientific field exploring the effects of sound on consciousness.

Entrainment

In *Healing Sounds* (1992), Jonathan Goldman discusses "entrainment" (14). He says that entrainment involves the ability of the more powerful rhythmic
vibration of one object to change the less powerful rhythmic vibration of another object and cause the second one to synchronize its rhythm with the first object. Goldman: "Through sound it is possible to change the rhythms of our brainwaves, as well as our heartbeat and respiration" (14). Many studies have been conducted on entrainment. If you put a dozen grandfather clocks in one room, all of the pendulums will entrain.

The four categories of brainwaves, Delta, Theta, Alpha, and Beta are equated to different states of consciousness. Brainwaves are based upon cycles per second (hertz or Hz). BioSonic Brain Tuners, available from SomaEnergetics are a great way to change the rhythm of our brainwaves. When the Fundamental Brain Tuner tuning fork is sounded with a Delta, Theta, Alpha, or Beta tuning fork the difference between the two tuning forks creates a binaural beat which is heard as a *pulsation*. The binaural beat gently signals the brain to shift into a different state of consciousness.

I once went to an Energy practitioner who did not know about the tuning forks but took an analysis of my voice. I spoke certain sounds into a vibration machine. The practitioner said there were *missing frequencies* in my voice analysis. I am so thankful I know how to fill in these missing frequencies today.

The six tones of the Solfeggio scale can fill in the gaps where the brain is still undeveloped and those blind spots of consciousness where we are not yet connected, neurologically. These original creative tones can operate in the Sacred Pause, to bring healing, health, and wholeness. We can change our health, we can change our world, we can reduce the chaos, relationship stresses, hostilities between nations, conflicts in religions, racism. All of these sociological phenomena emerge within humanity from the distorted vibrational frequencies of our contemporary world and I believe that every one can be reversed.

Process

Once again, I believe that the key word is the word "process." In quantum physics, scientists are beginning to realize that everything is process. Fritjof Capra in *The Tao of Physics* (2000)., elaborates on the tremendous shift in the thinking of the scientific community. He speaks in terms of a novel paradigm, one chacterized by mass movement away from "thinking in terms of structure, to thinking in terms of process. The processes that create sound into harmonious music are the same processes that govern all associating vibrations throughout the universe – and that includes everything that there is."(17)

In Christian Hummel's article "Sound, The Key To Ending War and Pollution" she asks:
> Did you know that the sounds of frogs, crickets and other insects and animals are necessary to maintaining the *bio-acoustic matrix*, or sonic envelope, of every delicate ecosystem? If the crickets stopped singing, the ecosystem where they lived would die. Dolphin sounds are responsible for the growth patterns of coral in reefs. According to

researcher Dan Carlson, a certain frequency in a bird's sound causes flowers to open. Native American Indians drummed to create the original sound we all heard when we were in the womb, the heartbeat vibration that brings balance and healing to the body and to the earth. (Hummel 2002)

Capra says,

> In the old paradigm, it was thought that there were fundamental structures, and then there were forces and mechanisms through which these interacted, which gave rise to processes. In the new paradigm, we think that *process is primary* (italics mine), that every structure we observe is a manifestation of an underlying process. (Capra 17)

As Einstein's Theory of Relativity originally stated: Mass is energy. There is no "matter." In this way, matter can be understood as songs that are so slow that they appear visible to the eye. Subatomic particles are not made of any material stuff. They are patterns of energy. Energy is associated with activity, with processes – all is a continuous dance of energy.

All is continual process. Material forms are continually being created and dissolved. We are the observers who determine what is created and what is dissolved. Did you get that part? Let me repeat the GOOD WORD for you: we are the observers who determine what is created and what is dissolved. We have to be involved in the process. We are a vital part of the process. Without us, there is no processing.

CHAPTER 9: DNA RESEARCH

Deoxyribonucleic Acid – DNA

When I saw that I had made a contract with Source to come to this free will planet, my continuing research made me realize that the code for the contract was in the etheric level of my DNA – also known as the *epigenome*. This word is derived from the Greek, *epi*, meaning "above or upon," and refers to the entire genome, including inactivated markers in the genetic (DNA) sequence. I wanted to know everything I could find out about DNA[1], or deoxyribonucleic acid. When this concept first occurred to me, I could not spell it; I could not even pronounce it. DNA was just beginning to come into the mass-mind consciousness. The first event that began to inform the public about DNA was the Human Genome Project, begun jointly in 1990 by the U.S. Department of Energy and National Institutes of Health. The second event that really put DNA on the tip of everyone's tongue was the O. J. Simpson trial. DNA became a household word after that. Now we regularly hear about DNA testing in the mass media.

Shortly after I had done this research about DNA, I booked a flight to Scottsdale, Arizona, to attend a DNA Meditation Activation Workshop by Robert Gerard, Ph.D. of the Oughten House Foundation.

Dr. Gerard has graciously given his information to the world, and I want to give him the most recognition I can for his

---

[1] DNA is a nucleic acid that carries the genetic information in the cell and is capable of self-replication and synthesis of RNA. DNA consists of two long chains of nucleotides twisted into a double helix and joined by hydrogen bonds between the complementary bases adenine and thymine or cytosine and guanine. The sequence of nucleotides determines individual hereditary characteristics. The American Heritage® Science Dictionary Copyright © 2005 by Houghton Mifflin Company. Published by Houghton Mifflin Company. All rights reserved

contribution to the planet's enlightenment. Dr. Gerard's message is this: "Our DNA, via the process of transcription by the RNA,[1] sends messages to the cell. The cells adapt by producing the necessary proteins, which in effect change the behavior of the cell function. Our internal DNA library, if you will, can sense its environment, change its structure, and send messages to reshape itself."[2] Gerard discusses a video documentary produced by Bruce Lipton titled *The Biology of Belief* (1999), which claims that awareness and perception are fundamental genetic determinants. Lipton clearly describes how evolution is distinctly modeled in the structure of the cell membrane and involves consciousness.

I totally resonated with Dr. Gerard's information. Combining my own research and intuition with experiences from Dr. Gerard's workshops, I began to conduct DNA Activation workshops while I continued to teach *A Course In Miracles*. I offered DNA Activation CD's produced by Visionary Music to students through my ministry. These CD's are available through my website.[3]

We know that two strands of DNA form a double helix, or spiral. Weak thermodynamic forces hold these two

---

[1] RNA is short for ribonucleic acid. The nucleic acid that is used in key metabolic processes for all steps of protein synthesis in all living cells and carries the genetic information of many viruses. Unlike double-stranded DNA, RNA consists of a single strand of nucleotides, and it occurs in a variety of lengths and shapes. RNA also differs from DNA in having the pyrimidine base uracil instead of thymine and in having ribose instead of deoxyribose in its sugar-phosphate backbone. In eukaryotes, RNA is produced in the cell nucleus. . . . Messenger RNA is RNA that carries genetic information from the cell nucleus to the structures in the cytoplasm (known as ribosomes) where protein synthesis takes place. . . . Ribosomal RNA is the main structural component of the ribosome. . . Transfer RNA is RNA that delivers the amino acids necessary for protein synthesis to the ribosomes. The American Heritage® Science Dictionary Copyright © 2005 by Houghton Mifflin Company. Published by Houghton Mifflin Company. All rights reserved.

[2] www.oughtenhouse.com; robertg@oughtenhouse.com.
[3] www.SomaEnergetics.com

polynucleotide chains together. Sequences of DNA letters (A, G, C & T – Adenine, Guanine, Cytosine, and Thymine – the substances found in nucleic acid in cells combine into complex sequences that make *words*, *sentences* and *paragraphs* that provide information and instructions to guide the formation of each cell. Each cell is encapsulated and has a membrane that holds everything inside the cell. The membrane is an oily outer boundary with receptors that seem to look at the material outside the cell to decide what will be allowed into the cell. DNA is inside this membrane. My belief is that soon we will know this membrane has consciousness.

The Dance of Shiva

According to Dr. Candace Pert, Ph.D. pharmacologist, in *Molecules of Emotion* (1999) it seems that these receptor molecules "respond to energy and chemical cues by vibrating. They wiggle, shimmy, and even hum as they bend and change. [. . .] They have roots that reach deep into the interior of the cell. " (22) These receptors on the outside of the cell act like scanners that hover on the membrane, dancing and vibrating, waiting to pick up messages carried by other vibrating little creatures that come cruising along.
In Hinduism, this rhythmic movement is called the Dance of Shiva which represents a delicate balance of creation and destruction, preservation and evolution – the death and rebirth of cells. Further, Fritjof Capra, in *The Tao of Physics* states:

> All things ... are aggregations of atoms that dance and by their movements produce sounds. When the rhythm of the dance changes, the sound it produces also changes... Each atom perpetually sings it song, and the sound, at every moment, creates dense and subtle forms. (1975, 242)

Receptors are proteins. They wait for the right chemical key to come along, to swim up to them in the extracellular fluid and to mount them by fitting into their keyholes in a process known as binding. My friends, this is sex on a molecular level. These little sex creatures are called ligands. As the ligand enters the keyhole, it tickles the molecule into changing its shape until – click, information enters the cell.

This information system is very complex. The information translation system, at the time of this writing, is still primarily a mystery. However, Dr. Pert suggests that "the mind is that which holds the network together, linking and coordinating the major systems and their organs and cells in an intelligently orchestrated symphony of life." (Pert, 185). There is an intelligence running things. You may have heard this called the "wisdom of the body." This is more proof of the mind-body connection. Dr. Pert continues, "A more dynamic description of this process might be two voices – ligand and receptor – striking the same note and producing a vibration that rings a doorbell to open the doorway to the cell. The message goes deep into the interior of the cell and can change the state of the cell dramatically." (24).

Living In The Field

This information blew my mind. While I was studying DNA, I continued to study quantum physics. In the sub-atomic world of particles and waves, theories of chaos, and the uncertainty principle, the architectural structure of Newton's Universe comes crashing down. What we believed to be fixed in stone is actually a continually moving and ever-changing Field of All Possibilities, all the time. Now, as I studied human DNA, I found that our DNA is not set in stone either. Apparently, nothing is.

Isn't this exciting? Life becomes an amazing adventure every single moment of every single hour of every single day. In November, 2006, *Discover Magazine* featured an article titled "DNA Is Not Your Destiny!" Even science is beginning to understand that DNA can be influenced by our feelings, attitudes, and intentions. We are living in an energy field; it is an electromagnetic field of strong and weak forces that constantly interact with themselves, and we are part of it. In fact, according to Heisenberg, without the observer, there is nothing to observe. We are the observer. We are critical to the overall operation of all things. Do you now see how important you are?

Pert says that the DNA information molecules: "...are the basic units of a language used by cells throughout our body to communicate across systems such as the endocrine, neurological, gastrointestinal and even the immune system. The musical hum of the receptors as they bind to their many ligands creates an integration of structure and function that allows the body to run smoothly and intelligently." (27).

Inside our bodies there is music playing. All of our internal organs are humming away. Each organ hums at a certain vibration and all of the cells of the body are humming together, making a virtual cellular symphony of music. If one organ gets out of tune, we do not feel well. We get uncomfortable and dis-eased. Others, such as Barbara Hero also advocate this view of the body's symphony. Hero, in particular, has done the research to determine the frequency of every organ in the body. She makes this information available to everyone, via her website, where one can find a list of these frequencies for further consideration and to fuel your imagination.[1]

Then, why do we not just tune that organ back up to its original hum? How can we do this? Read On. This is process. You are getting to know process.

Turning the Switch On

Through my foray into DNA, I learned that the assembly instructions for the human body are contained in human DNA, as read and interpreted by the RNA. At each of

---

[1] Refer to http://www.greatdreams.com/hertz.htm for more information

twenty sites on the DNA, there are codons, binary switches, meaning that they can be either ON or OFF. These twenty switches, which are believed to be ON, produce humans with the characteristics we know. An additional forty sites have switches that have always, or for a long time, been in the OFF position. Many believe that if some or all of these switches could be flipped ON, an entirely new type of human would be produced. In particular terms, this new human – homoluminous – would be characterized by mastery over illness, disease, linear time and death. In short, this new human would be the embodiment of a complete union of body, mind, and spirit.

Some believe that this is now happening. Contemporary genetics informs us that there is a possibility of 64 codons within the scope of what is characterized as human. Many metaphysical social theorists are speculating that some of the children coming to earth today have 21, 22, 23, or 24 codons in operation. Often they have been judged ADHD. Although some may have legitimate physiological pre-conditions associated with their birth, it is entirely possible that the large majority are just "wired" differently. We do not have the systems or procedures to know how to deal with these children, so we typically drug them. However, I believe these are the kids who have the answers to all of our problems. They are the next step in our evolution. We should be listening to them, not drugging them.[1]

Who are these new humans? What could flip their switches to the ON position? I believe it is the new frequencies contained in the higher energy coming upon our planet earth right now. Not only that, I believe with all of my heart that we can tickle these switches and get them turned on within ourselves. I believe we can awaken the part of ourselves that is asleep. I believe we can make this next step in our evolution and become self-empowered, walking in our own knowledge and revelation, freely giving to the whole of Creation that part of us that is unique and

---

[1] (Refer to http://www.indigochild.net for additional information)

wonderful. One way we can begin the process is by learning how to use the vibratory patterns produced by the six ancient sounds of the original Solfeggio tuning forks.

There are 35,000 genes in each human DNA molecule, made up of three billion chemical bases arranged in precise sequences. Remember, these sequences of letters (A, G, C, T) make up the alphabet of DNA, combining into their versions of words, sentences, and paragraphs. They operate like the zero-and-one binary code that computers understand. Following are some mind-blowing statistics about DNA. Each strand of the double helix is 3 feet long. Within the nucleus of a cell, DNA folds into a space of a few thousandths of a millimeter. Moreover, so far, we only use 3% of it to regulate the human system.

Now, with the advent of quantum physics, we know that the observer is as important to the formation and function of life at the cellular level as the energy of life itself. There is a Divine Master at the keyboard of the original software program that created you. That Divine Master has turned the process of your life and your health over to YOU!

Misspelled DNA

As I studied everything I could find about the DNA, it seemed that if we came into life with certain pre-dispositions to diseases or weaknesses, then we had some misspelled words in our DNA. The sequences of the letters could be out-of-order. An out-of-order paragraph could make a weak heart, or a misspelled word of DNA could make a hammertoe. I thought about all of the disparities and disfigurements of the human body. If everything is dictated and influenced by our DNA, then, in some people – maybe in all people – there might be mistakes in the original DNA sequencing.

When sick, many people typically go to a western doctor. We are asked about family members and how they lived, and how they died. Our medical chart includes our family history of pre-dispositions to diseases that are believed to be hereditary, such as heart trouble, cancer, or diabetes. This makes me think of a verse in the *Bible*, that reads, "[...] visiting the iniquity of the fathers upon the children, and upon the children's children, unto the third and to the fourth generation." (Exodus 34:7) It has been said that "Sin is coming short of the Glory of God." In the past, our parents and grandparents lived their lives short of the Glory of God. They did not know who they really were. So those misfirings of their DNA were encoded into the next generation's DNA and passed down between ancestors. As descendents, we believe we have the chance of having heart trouble because our father or our grandfather died of heart trouble, so we "inherit" the weakness. Belief manifests on the cellular level of everyday body reality.

Apparently, genetic predisposition is not the TRUTH. Nothing is set in stone. Is it possible that we can be set free of inherited DNA weaknesses? Carl Sagan and old Newtonian science say that we only use 3% of our DNA and the rest is gibberish. That means 97% is considered DNA gibberish, or "junk." The 97% was allegedly left after we evolved into a human being.[1]

Nevertheless, if 97% of our DNA is genetic gibberish, in the end we still have 97% of DNA that has not been used yet. It has yet to be evolved, explored, and experienced. It is as if God said, "I'll give you 3% of your mind that you can use for anything you want. You can try anything and do anything you want. You can believe anything you want to. I know you will start all kinds of religions and literally try to build yourself a staircase to heaven. But I am closing your womb of consciousness to the other 97%." In other words, outside conditioning cannot penetrate 97% of the genetic material held within each human cell. Not by culture, society, religion, education, not even our genetic information can penetrate this 97% of untapped, unused, pure potential of the human being. I believe this untapped 97% is what we

---

[1] Carl Sagan & Ann Druyan Shadows of Forgotten Ancestors (1993)

have called "Spirit" in the hierarchies of religion, but is really the untapped part of God that is in us and ready to BE US.

The great theologian, Pierre Teilhard de Chardin, SJ, said (1881-1955), "We are not humans in a physical body trying to have a spiritual experience, but we are spirits trying to have a human experience." Therefore, it would seem that we have had only about 3% of the human experience at this point.

I now believe that when I used to "speak in tongues" while preaching, I was literally activating parts of my 97% genetic gibberish. There were times that we saw what we called "Miracles." Blind eyes could see, deaf ears could hear, and the crippled walked. I cannot deny that these healings and miracles took place – I just never understood what was happening or why it only took place with some people and not others until I came across this information about the DNA. Part of the 97% of the genetic gibberish can be activated. One example of this activation taking form is as a miracle healing. I believe that today I can live my life as a miracle. We only call it a miracle because we do not understand the process. God does not see it as a miracle. God just sees it as normal behavior, normal life. I believe we can become humans who operate in the full 100% of our genetic material.

Let Us Move On

As we move from belief in genetic disposition and concepts like Body, Soul, and Spirit, dividing us into fragmented beings, we move beyond physical diagnosis into the new area of quantum physics. In this new area, where consciousness is seen as a Unified Field and where Everything is Everything Else (also known as the Theory of Everything[1] or T.O.E.), there are no boundaries. There is no

---

[1] - Ellis, John (1986), "The superstring: theory of everything, or of nothing?", Nature 323: 595–598.

"this" or "that," no "you" or "me." It is a pure Field of Awareness. My own perception has now changed from genetics to energetics. I now realize that we are not meant to ignore our physiology, but rather that it is a pathway to learn to tune our body and get it operating at the specific frequencies that each part requires.

As one of the original developers of therapeutic tuning forks "tuned" to the same frequencies as the ancient Solfeggio tones, my dedication, commitment and belief in the power of these ancient frequencies has led me to the development and founding of SomaEnergetics. Much thought went into this name, combining the Greek word *soma*, meaning "body", with *energetics*, to capture in one word the wholistic idea of the body as a vibrant energy field. I firmly believe that these sacred tones actually serve as a "vibrational bridge" to wholistic re-integration of the physical, mental, emotional, and spiritual aspects of the individual. The SomaEnergetics workshops have been created to teach and empower people to discover and use these long lost frequencies for self healing and for assisting others in achieving their health and wellness goals.

I encourage you to let go of all thoughts of separation that divide you from the universe, the cosmos, and others. Traditionally, SPIRIT seemed to be something detached from us, something we did not have and could only get through systems of religions. Remember, as Teilhard deChardin said so well, "We are not human beings trying to attain a spiritual experience, but rather, we are spiritual beings having a human experience." And with that deep and great Truth, I make my call to you. Come with me and go forth into the realms of health and happiness. Learn about the tuning forks tuned to the ancient tones of the original Solfeggio. Take them into your life. Balance your life. And then, be a channel of this Truth and Energy to the whole Earth. I invite you to become a Co-Worker with me to restore human consciousness to its full power and potential, the realization of what Mark Twain so beautifully described when he wrote:

Inherently, each one of us has the substance within to achieve whatever our goals and dreams define. What is missing from each of us are the training, education, knowledge and insight to utilize what we already have.

David Hulse, D.D.

APPENDIX A

Numbers Chapter 7 KJV

Verse: 1st 3 are highlighted to show beginning of pattern

12 **(3)** And he that offered his offering the ***first day*** was Nahshon the son of Amminadab, of the tribe of Judah
13 And his offering was ***one silver charger***, the weight thereof was an hundred and thirty shekels, one silver bowl of seventy shekels, after the shekel of the sanctuary; both of them were full of fine flour mingled with oil for a meat offering
14 One spoon of ***ten shekels*** of gold, full of incense
15 One young bullock, one ram, one lamb of the first year, for a burnt offering
16 One kid of the goats for a sin offering
17 And for a sacrifice of peace offerings, two oxen, five rams, five he goats, five lambs of the first year: this was the offering of Nahshon the son of Amminadab.
18 **(9)** On the ***second day*** Nethaneel the son of Zuar, prince of Issachar, did offer
19 He offered for his offering ***one silver charger***, the weight whereof was an hundred and thirty shekels, one silver bowl of seventy shekels, after the shekel of the sanctuary; both of them full of fine flour mingled with oil for a meat offering
20 One spoon of gold of ***ten shekels***, full of incense
21 One young bullock, one ram, one lamb of the first year, for a burnt offering
22 One kid of the goats for a sin offering
23 And for a sacrifice of peace offerings, two oxen, five rams, five he goats, five lambs of the first year: this was the offering of Nethaneel the son of Zuar.
24 **(6)** On the ***third day*** Eliab the son of Helon, prince of the children of Zebulun, did offer
25 His offering was ***one silver charger***, the weight whereof was an hundred and thirty shekels, one silver bowl of seventy shekels, after the shekel of the sanctuary; both of them full of fine flour mingled with oil for a meat offering
26 One golden spoon of ***ten shekels***, full of incense
27 One young bullock, one ram, one lamb of the first year, for a burnt offering
28 One kid of the goats for a sin offering
29 And for a sacrifice of peace offerings, two oxen, five rams, five he goats, five lambs of the first year: this was the offering of Eliab the son of Helon.

Continues for the rest of chapter 7 with the same pattern repeating…

WORKS CITED

Apel, Willi. 1958. *Gregorian Chant*. Bloomington, Indiana: Indiana University Press.

Ash, Steven. 2001. *Sacred Drumming*. New York: Sterling.

Beaulieu, John. 1995. *Music and Sound in the Healing Arts*. Barrytown, NY: Station Hill Press.

Berendt, Joachim-Ernst t. 1991. The World Is Sound: Nada Brahma: Music and the Landscape of Consciousness. Rochester, Vermont: Destiny Books.

Braden, Greg. 1997. *Awakening to Zero Point*. Gallatin, TN: Sacred Spaces Ancient Wisdom

Brennan, Barbara. 1988. *Hands of Light*. New York: Bantam.

Byrne, Rhonda. 2006. The Secret. Hillsboro, OR: Atria Books/Beyond Words.

Capra, Fritjof. 2000. *The Tao of Physics*. Boston, MA: Shambhala Publications, Inc.

Chladni, Ernst. 1989. *Sound and Vibration Magazine*, November.

Chopra, Deepak. 1992. *Higher Self (Audiocassette Series)*. Niles, IL: Nightingale Conant.

Clay, Gary and Verna Clay. *Solfa Sound Training Manual*. http://www.solfasound.org.

Conforto, Guiliana. 1998, *Man's Cosmic Game*. **Edizioni Noesis.**

Critchlow, Keith. 1982. *Time Stands Still*. Edinburgh, Scotland: Floris Books.

Doty, David. 1993. *The Just Intonation Primer*. San Francisco, CA: Just Intonation Network.

Dubro, Peggy and David Lapierre. 2002. *Elegant Empowerment*. Sedona, Arizona: Platinum Publishing House.

Fry, Christopher. 1951. *A Sleep of Prisoners, A Play*. London: Oxford University Press.

Gerber, Richard. 2001. *Vibrational Medicine* . Rochester, Vermont: Bear & Company.

Goldman, Jonathan. 2002. *Healing Sounds: The Power of Harmonics*. Rochester, Vermont: Healing Arts Press.

Guzzetta, Cathie E. 1991. Music Therapy: Nursing the Music of the Soul, in Music: Physician for the Times to Come, Wheaton, IL: Quest Books.

Horowitz, Leonard. 1999. *Healing Codes for the Biological Apocalypse*. Sandpoint, ID: Tetrahedron Publishing Group.

Hulse, David. 1999. Take Another Look:
A Scriptural Review of Traditional Christian Doctrines.
www.lightwithin.com.

Hummel, Christan. 2002 "Sound, The Key to Ending War and Pollution?" *Sound Magazine*, November.

Hurtak, J.J. 1977. The Book of Knowledge: *The Keys of Enoch*. Los Gatos, CA: Academy for Future Science.

Isacoff, Stuart. 2001. Temperament: The idea that Solved Music's Greatest Riddle. New York: Alfred A. Knopf.

Jenny, Hans. 2001. Cymatics: A Study of Wave Phenomena & Vibration. Newmarket, NH: MACROomedia.

Lipton, Bruce. 1999. *The Biology of Belief (Audio)* Louisville, CO: Sounds True.

Lawler, Robert. 1982. *Sacred Geometry.* New York: Crossroad.

Logue, Christopher. 1969. "Come to the Edge", *New Numbers*. London: Jonathan Cape Ltd.

Luckman, Sol. 2005. *Conscious Healing.* http://www.booklocker.com.

Marciniak, Barbara. 1994. *Earth: Pleiadian Keys to the Living Library*. Rochester, Vermont: Bear & Company.

Myss, Caroline. 2001. *The Energetics of Healing (VHS)*. http://shop.soundstrue.com.

Narby, Jeremy. 1999. *The Cosmic Serpent*. New York: Tarcher.

Payne, R.E. 2003. *The End of All Disease.* Bloomington, IA: AuthorHouse.

Pearce, Joseph Chilton. 2002. *Biology of Transcendence*. Rochester VT: **Park Street Press.**

Pert, Candace. 1999. *Molecules of Emotion.* : New York: Simon & Schuster.

Pond, Dale et al. 1995. *Universal Laws Never Before Revealed:Keely's Secrets*. Santa Fe, NM: The Message Company.

Rees, Martin. 1999. *Just Six Numbers*. NewYork: Basic Books.

Schookman, Helen. 2007. *A Course in Miracles*. Mill Valley, CA. ; **Foundation for Inner Peace.**

Starkman GD and D.J. Schwarz. 2005. "Is the Universe Out of Tune?" *Scientific American* Vol. 293 Number 2: 48 – 55.

Talbot, Michael .1992. *The Holographic Universe*. New York: **Harper Perennial.**

Watters, Ethan. November, 2006. "DNA is not Your Destiny," *Discover Magazine*.

Wolf, Fred A. 2000. *Mind into Matter: A New Alchemy of Science and Spirit*. Needham, MA : Moment Point Press.

Zukav, Gary . 1999. *The Seat of the Soul.* New York: Simon & Schuster.

WEBSITES CITED

Conforto, Giuliana.
http://www.giulianaconforto.it/English/home.Eng.htm

Doty, David . The Just Intonation Primer.
http://www.justintonation.net/primer2.html

Franklin, Ruth. Good Vibrations. The New Republic Online.
http://www.powells.com/review/2001_12_13.html).

Gann, Kyle. Just Intonation Explained..
http://www.kylegann.com/tuning.html>).

Hummel, Christian. The Power of Sound.
http://earthtransitions.com/Alchemy-of-Sound/The-Power-of-Sound.html

The Tomatis Method. http://tomatis.com/ 2001-2008

Ut Queant Laxis.
http://en.wikipedia.org/wiki/Ut_queant_laxis

About the Author...

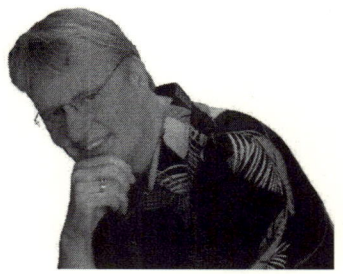

David Hulse, D.D. combines his over four decades of experience as a motivational speaker with years of research in metaphysics, science, sound and spirituality to bring you a unique and empowering journey. At the turn of the century, this unique background served as the catalyst for David's accelerating interest and research into the lost frequencies of the Ancient Solfeggio.

These ancient sound frequencies were apparently used in Ancient Gregorian Chants, that church authorities say were lost centuries ago. The chants and their special tones were believed to impart tremendous spiritual blessings, when sung. David's further research then led him into the dynamics of sound, and its influence on the etheric/physical interface. As a result, he felt led to develop tuning forks that are tuned to the frequencies of the Ancient Solfeggio.

Today, David believes that these Ancient, Sacred Tones actually serve as a "vibrational bridge" to holistically re-integrate the physical, mental, emotional and spiritual aspects of the individual, as well as all of Humanity—collectively. His diverse background allows him to speak on a wide range of topics. By using the deep metaphysical meanings found in the scriptures, the psychology of A Course In Miracles, and exploring the enlightened discoveries coming from new science about Light and Sound.

David's presentations incorporate science, psychology and world religions in a unique combination that is easy to understand. This uniqueness allows him to reach diverse audiences seeking a path of enlightenment and his ability to gather fragments of truth from many different disciplines and tap into present truth, helps bring all of your experiences up to now into focus.

David Hulse, D.D. is the original Developer of the SomaEnergetics Energy Balancing Techniques utilizing the Ancient Solfeggio Tuning Forks. He holds a Doctorate of Divinity Degree from the American Institute of Holistic Theology.

The Solfeggio Frequencies in Water Crystals

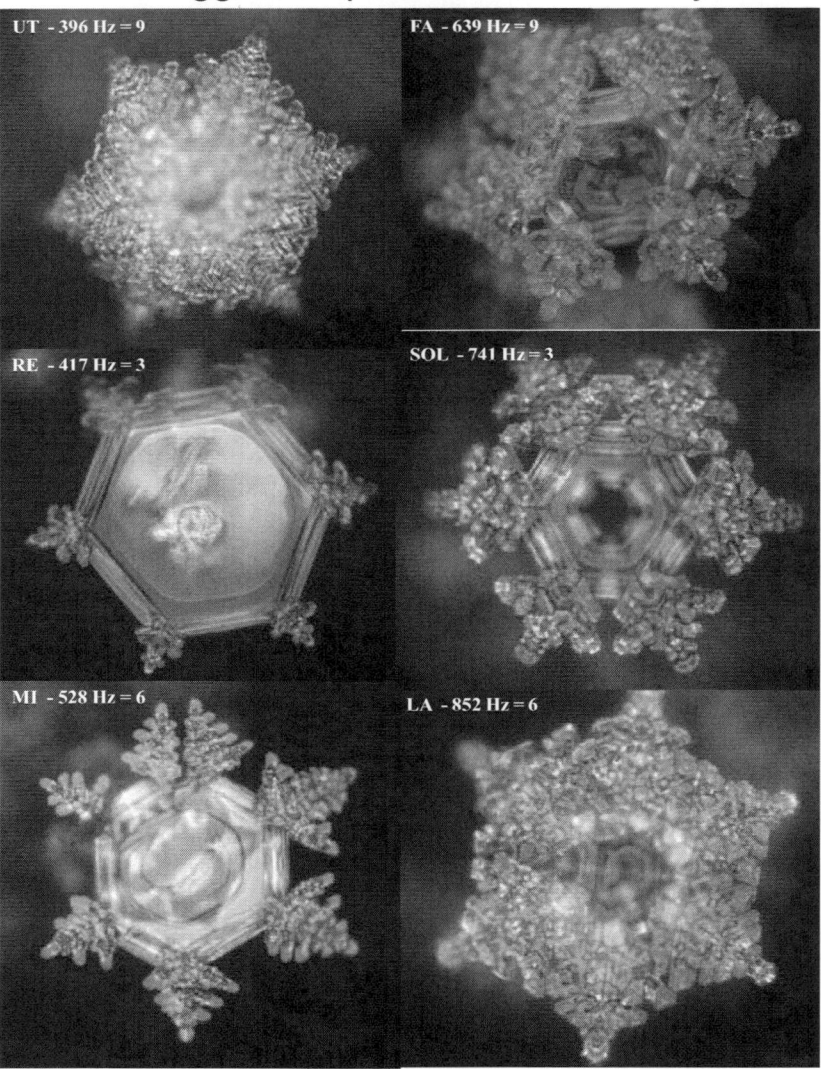

These were discovered by Dr. Edmund Gergerian and passed onto David Hulse.
From Jay Emmanuel's site http://powerofharmony.tripod.comfreezing_water.htm

Made in the USA
San Bernardino, CA
06 April 2013